A woman's diagnose-it-yourself guide to health

Dr Sarah Jarvis,
Dr Keith Hopcroft
and Dr Alistair Moulds

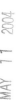

OXFORD

UNIVERSITY PRESS

OXFORD

UNIVERSITY PRESS

Great Clarendon Street, Oxford OX2 6DP, UK

Oxford University Press is a department of the University of Oxford.
It furthers the University's objective of excellence in research, scholarship,
and education by publishing worldwide in

Oxford New York

Athens Auckland Bangkok Bogotá Buenos Aires Calcutta
Cape Town Chennai Dar es Salaam Delhi Florence Hong Kong Istanbul
Karachi Kuala Lumpur Madrid Melbourne Mexico City Mumbai
Nairobi Paris São Paulo Singapore Taipei Tokyo Toronto Warsaw

with associated companies in
Berlin Ibadan

Oxford is a registered trade mark of Oxford University Press
in the UK and in certain other countries

Published in the United States
by Oxford University Press, Inc., New York

© S. Jarvis, K. Hopcroft, A. Moulds, 2000

British Library Cataloguing in Publication Data
Data available

Library of Congress Cataloging in Publication Data

1 3 5 7 9 10 8 6 4 2

ISBN 0 19 263260 4
Typeset by
J & L Composition Ltd, Filey, North Yorkshire
Printed in Great Britain on acid free paper by
Biddles Ltd., Guildford & King's Lynn

Contents

Introduction

We are a nation obsessed with our health – for women, at least, the saying 'You can never be too rich or too thin' might be translated into 'You can never be too informed about health and calories'.

But we are also a nation obsessed with time – or rather, the lack of it. Every year, more of the working population is made up of working women – just 60 years ago, the figure was four million, while today it's nearer 13 million. These days, we're more likely to hear women complaining that they need a wife rather than a money-off token for washing powder. Quite simply, the traditional model of the wife who cleans the whole house daily and still has time to kill before she collects her little darlings from school just doesn't cut it.

Part of the myth is that once the kids are off her hands, the average woman has plenty of free time to spend on herself. Well, in your dreams. In a recent survey almost 80% of the women interviewed felt they never had enough time to spend on themselves, and two-thirds regularly felt too exhausted even to have sex.

But having better things to do than sit around in the GP's waiting room, dreaming of the wholesome but tasty dinner you're going to serve your man, doesn't mean you don't need sound health advice. If anything, with all the added stresses women are under, we reckon you need accurate, reader-friendly information more than ever.

Not that there isn't plenty of sensible stuff out there. It's just that for the most part, all the best information seems to be about conditions you don't have – and if it is what you want, it's scattered all over the place in the shape of odd leaflets, that you can never seem to find when you want to. That's where this book comes in.

We'd like to let you in on a little medical trade secret. About 90% of the information doctors use to work out what's wrong with you comes from the history – what you tell the doctor. Contrary to popular belief, examining you usually just serves to confirm what the doc already knows from that chat before you jumped up on the couch. It also explains why the doc can sort out so many problems over the phone.

What we're aiming to do with this diagnose-it-yourself guide is to give *you* the information you need to make easy, reliable, step-by-step diagnoses. Once you've worked out what you've got, we tell you what to do about it. This way, you don't need to spend unnecessary hours waiting to see your doc, but you won't ignore something that might need treatment.

We're not going to pretend that the book will get it right 100% of the time. No one knows better than we do that illnesses don't read textbooks, and that sometimes they show themselves in ways they're not supposed to. That's why we

tend to err on the side of caution – if your symptoms don't quite fit, or if they don't settle down by themselves, we would always advise you to get them checked out. But for the most part, reading the information in this book carefully and sensibly will give you a pretty clear idea of what action – if any – you need to take.

One final point: we're aware that doctors can be male as well as female. We've used the female form throughout to avoid wordiness, and because so many women choose to go to a woman doctor.

Sarah Jarvis
Keith Hopcroft
Alistair Moulds

October 2000

How to use this book

Part One, 'Staying on Top', gives no-nonsense tips on getting medical help when you need it and making the most of seeing your GP. Part Three, 'Having it all', looks at lifestyle and how it affects health – we've deliberately avoided a preachy approach in this particular section because (a) We think life is about quality as much as quantity; (b) Some traditionally 'frowned-upon' activities aren't half as bad as originally thought and may even be good for you and (c) We don't want you to bin the book.

The final section, 'Don't get pregnant...but if you do' gives the low-down on contraception and what to do if you're planning to take the plunge into the world of nappies and baby-puke.

Sandwiched between Parts One and Three is the 'diagnose-it-yourself' guide: virtually all the common symptoms you're likely to suffer are included. So here's how you become your own doctor.

Step one **Check your age**

This book is aimed at 'young women', who we arbitrarily define as women in the 15–45 age bracket. The older you are (and particularly if you're above 45) the greater the likelihood that a symptom you're suffering might have a significant cause – or a cause linked to areas we don't cover in detail (such as the menopause). So although those of you over 45 might find the flow charts useful and interesting, you should not rely on them, and you should have a lower threshold for seeing your GP.

Step two **Find your symptom**

The symptoms are arranged in alphabetical order. If a quick flick through the contents draws a blank, use the index to find the page you need.

Step three **Follow the chart**

A series of simple yes/no questions should lead you to the diagnosis. Each diagnosis has extra clues to help you check you've got it right. Every so often, you might come across these logos: ⚠ and ⚠. The first means you'll need to see your GP sharpish, the second that you need urgent medical help. They're on the charts to get important information across quickly and clearly, and to make the pages prettier.

Step four **Find out how likely your diagnosis is and what it means**

The information accompanying the flow chart gives more detail about your problem and explains what you should do about it. Note: if you've ended up with a 'Longer shot' diagnosis then either you've got an unusual problem or you've got it wrong. It's worth thinking again and trying another run through the flow chart.

But what happens if you have a number of symptoms which you think are probably linked in some way? Easy. Simply select the one that's bothering you most and follow the steps outlined above. This will give you the likely diagnosis. You can then go through the same process with the next most bothersome symptom to see if the diagnosis for this one matches the first, and so on. For example, if you're suffering from headaches, problems sleeping and an uptight feeling then you're likely to find that the common thread is stress and tension. If your self diagnoses don't seem to have any real link then either you've made a mistake somewhere along the line– so use the book to try again - or you may actually have more than one problem.

That's it. Young woman heal thyself.

Part One

Staying on top

Well, it's official. Among the many things girls are better at than blokes (remembering birthdays, washing out the bath, communicating – the list is endless!), it seems they're also better at going to see their GP. They certainly go more often, with gynae problems, contraception, smears, and antenatal checks giving more reasons to go, so the average female becomes very familiar with the inside of a GP's waiting room.

However, this doesn't really make the prospect of a trip to the GP any less stressful. It's not as simple as wafting into the consulting room with a problem and wafting out with a magic potion – you have to get an appointment, fit it into your busy schedule, and get to the surgery on time before you even reach the doctor herself. All of which, in these hectic days, is more liable to make you neurotic than a bad bout of PMT.

Of course you don't need to go and see your GP for absolutely everything – far from it. There are dozens of alternative sources of advice and treatment out there, but it can be tricky trying to work out where to go for what. Here, then, are a few pointers about who else may be able to help.

Your local chemist. These days, pharmacists are far more than peddlars of vitamins and indigestion remedies. They're highly trained and can offer advice about a wide range of ailments, as well as telling you whether or not you need to see your GP. Some very effective treatments which have, until fairly recently, only been available on prescription, can now be bought from your local pharmacy. These include various treatments for thrush; ibuprofen (an anti-inflammatory drug for aches, strains, and period pains); hydrocortisone 1% cream (for eczema); and various powerful indigestion treatments and anti-diarrhoea remedies. Most of these aren't available in the supermarket – and the pharmacist will only give them after he has asked you some questions to make sure they are right for you.

For some conditions, cystitis for example, your pharmacist will be able to offer a treatment that may not cure your condition but will at least relieve your symptoms until you can get to your GP. For other minor conditions, such as tickly coughs, tummy bugs, and colds, the pharmacist should certainly be your first port of call. You can also buy very accurate pregnancy tests there – they can often give you the answer to the BIG question on the day you miss your period!

Casualty. The great advantages of casualty are that you don't need an appointment and you can turn up when you want. The downsides are that the queues are often horrendous, there's usually a fair selection of noisy drunks waiting to try and chat you up and, even when you are seen, you may be referred back to your GP with an embarrassing slap on the wrist for using the department inappropriately.

Problems which should be taken to casualty

NB   This is for guidance only – and there's nothing to stop you taking a quick look at the appropriate flow chart in this book if you're in doubt.

- significant injury to limbs or trunk (e.g. possible broken bone, a cut which might need stitching)
- head injury (if a severe bump, knocked out for any length of time, loss of memory, or drowsiness)
- an eye injury
- a knee injury with sudden swelling (i.e. within minutes)
- all but the mildest burns
- severe chest pain
- severe shortness of breath
- severe, constant pain in the abdomen
- sudden, severe headache with drowsiness and/or vomiting
- vomiting blood (except a few streaks after a lot of retching)
- any overdose (deliberate or accidental)
- poisoning
- any loss of consciousness (other than a faint, or a fit if you're known to be epileptic and you recover from it quickly)
- inability to pass urine (at all)
- feeling depressed to the point of suicide

So how do you know whether you should be there at all? Easy – just remember that it's also called an 'accident and emergency department'. If you are 'an accident or an emergency', you're in the right place. If you definitely aren't, hide your face in one of those four-year-old copies of *Hello* in the waiting room so no one recognizes you before you can sneak out and seek more appropriate help. If you're not sure, you could consult the information box below, or ring the casualty department or GP's surgery before you leave home to find out where you should go.

Family planning clinics. Most big towns and cities have family planning clinics, where you can get contraception, pregnancy tests, and smears. The advantages are likely to include evening appointments, female doctors, and little chance of running into a friend of your Mum's. You can look up your nearest in the phone book – but remember, the doctor there won't have all your medical records, and you may find yourself being referred back to your GP if you go in with anything other than a routine request for contraception or a smear.

Sexually transmitted disease clinics. These are known by a variety of names ('clap clinic', 'special clinic', department of genito-urinary medicine) and most local hospitals have one. These days, they aren't populated exlcusively by old men in dirty raincoats, you don't need an appointment, and they are extremely careful about confidentiality. It's especially important for you to get yourself seen to quickly if you think you might have a sexually transmitted disease. Some of these types of germs can block your fallopian tubes, causing later problems with infertility, even if they cause little in the way of symptoms at the time – and even if getting pregnant is the last thing on your mind just now, that may not always be the case!

So how can you tell that you might have a sexually transmitted disease? You might get a smelly vaginal discharge, abnormal vaginal bleeding, low abdominal pain, or pain when you make love. For more information, see the sections on 'Abnormal or irregular vaginal bleeding' (p. 16), 'Vaginal discharge' (p. 148), and 'Lower abdominal pain – recurrent' (p. 94). If you think there is any chance you have a sexually transmitted disease, you should phone your local hospital for the opening times of the clinic and get yourself there as soon as you can – usually within a day or two. If your symptoms are really bad, you might want to get help sooner than the time of the next clinic, in which case you could call your GP – but she may want to send you to the clinic later anyway for specialist tests and 'contact tracing' to see where you or your partner picked up the infection.

The telephone. It's a fairly safe bet that, whatever your problem, somewhere in the country there's at least one person sitting by the telephone waiting for you to ring. The problem, of course, is finding the right number to call. This may be harder than it seems (for instance, there are hundreds of groups offering advice to people with alcohol problems or their families – but in most phone books they're listed, not under A for Alcohol services, but under D for Drug and alcohol services). As well as local advice lines, many self-help groups have national advice lines run by volunteers with plenty of experience of the relevant condition. Now the government is getting in on the act too. **NHS Direct (0845 4647)** is a new 24-hour helpline, manned by trained nurses, which is being developed nationally to offer advice on medical problems and NHS services.

Of course, your GP has a telephone as well, and you may be able to avoid the hassle of going to see her by using it. This isn't just when you need a certificate or have run out of your Pill the day before your holiday – she can give you advice on many ailments too. Most GPs have certain times when they take calls – look in your practice leaflet or ask your GP's receptionist – or they may ring you back if you leave a message with the receptionist.

The Internet. The great thing about the Internet is that with a computer, a phone line, and a modem you can access it any time, and there is a huge amount of information out there. But this has its disadvantages too. Sifting through the billion bytes of data to find what you really need can be a nightmare. Unless you have spent the last 10 years on the planet Zorg, you can't have failed to notice that the Net is the place to be – for all sorts of nutcases and cranks as well as for genuine experts. Since the Internet is entirely unpoliced, it's a magic opportunity for people with strongly held views or an eye to the main chance to get their views across on a huge range of subjects. That's not to say that the Internet doesn't have a lot to offer – it can be a great opportunity to find out about new advances in disease management all over the world. Just try to stick to reputable websites (such as registered websites from universities or research institutes) and be aware that not everything you read on the Internet should be taken as gospel.

Complementary therapists. Complementary therapists seem to be multiplying at the same rate as mobile phones, and need to be chosen just as carefully. In these days of self-awareness and self-help, it's hardly surprising that the concept of 'natural' healing can be very appealing. The problem is that, as with the Internet, there are a lot of cranks and fakes out there mixed in with the genuine articles.

Some complementary therapies now have their own accredited body, which checks up on it's members' qualifications and can strike them off its register if they behave unprofessionally. Unfortunately, for most of the complementary therapies, membership of these organizations is voluntary, and if members are struck off they can still keep practising.

Some of the complementary therapies can appear very effective (osteopathy and acupuncture, for instance), some aren't going to do you much harm even if they don't work (aromatherapy and reflexology) – and if you think they'll do you good, they probably will. This is commonly known as the placebo effect (or perhaps 'mind over matter'), and there's nothing like parting with fifty quid a session to concentrate the mind on the need to get better! Far more worrying are 'alternative' rather than 'complementary' practitioners, who believe that their treatment will only work if you give up your conventional treatment. This can be bad news and such advice should never be followed blindly.

On the whole, we are pretty sceptical about a lot of alternative or complementary therapies, but if you do want to go down this route, try and check out the therapist thoroughly first – personal recommendation is always useful, but so are details of qualifications and professional registration.

Going private. There aren't many private GPs around but there are more and more private 'walk-in' clinics, which may be useful if you are pushed for time and they are close to your work. Remember, though, that as with family planning clinics, these doctors won't have your full medical records and are unlikely to offer any continuity of care. The one thing they will offer, of course, is a pretty hefty bill!

The receptionist at your doctor's surgery. Long gone are the days when the receptionist took pride in keeping attendances down by terrorizing anyone brave enough to try and gain access to the hallowed portals of the GP's consulting room. These days they may still try to direct you away from the doctor, but their tactics are more subtle and often very appropriate. They may offer you a practice leaflet which tells you how to get the most out of the system, or point you to the practice nurse or even the nurse practitioner. Whatever you want from the GP's surgery, it's worth remembering that the receptionist probably knows how to get it – so it's well worth getting her on your side.

This book. The flow charts and the explanatory blurb will help you work out when you can self-treat and when you really need to see an expert.

So what if you have decided you really do need to see your GP? How do you go about it without wasting too much precious time and without losing your temper and your sanity? And once you're there, how do you make the most of it?

How to see your GP

These days, most GPs' surgeries run an appointment system, and you can make an appointment just by ringing up. However, even this seemingly simple process can be frustrating. Here are a few useful tips:

- Try not to ring first thing in the morning, especially on a Monday – the phone lines will probably be jammed solid.

- Try to book an appointment a fews days in advance if you can. Of course, this may not be possible for urgent problems, but the more notice you give, the better your prospects of getting an appointment with the doctor you want, at a time you really want, especially for popular slots like the first and last of the day.

- If your doc always tends to run late, it may be worth trying to book the first appointment of morning or evening surgery – most GPs start their surgeries on time, but they may gradually fall further and further behind as the session goes on.

- Find out if your surgery runs any late evening or Saturday morning surgeries for busy punters. Bear in mind, though, that Saturday morning surgeries may be reserved for emergencies, so check before you turn up wanting a repeat prescription for acne lotion.

- If your doc is usually heavily booked up and you need to see someone fairly soon, make it clear that you are happy to see any doctor at the practice – some will have free slots much sooner than others. If you need to consult about an ongoing problem, though, don't forget that your own doctor will know more about your case, so it may be worth waiting unless the problem is obviously urgent.

- These days, most practices have at least one female doctor (and a few have nothing but), so you should have a choice of whether or not you see one. It is worth checking, though, before you sign up as a patient because even if you don't mind who you see for most things, there may be some female conditions you'd feel happier confiding to another woman. A few practices run personal lists, which means they insist on you seeing the same doc for everything – which might be an issue if your registered doc is a man. Bear in mind, though, that even an all-male practice is likely to have a nurse providing special services like family planning or smears.

- Ask when you first register (or at least before you get ill) about the practice policy for seeing 'emergencies'. Most practices will have flexibility built into their system so that urgent problems can be seen the same day. Remember, though, that you are far more likely to have to spend ages in the waiting room if you don't have a routine booked appointment – so take a good book if you don't want to resort to reading back issues of *Fly-fisher Monthly*.

- You do have a right to be seen urgently if you have an urgent problem. Don't forget, though, that many docs won't deal with anything except the urgent problem at that time and may ask you to book another appointment for the non-urgent bits.

- If you don't feel your problem can wait for a routine appointment, say so when you first speak to a receptionist. Likewise, if you don't feel your problem is being taken seriously, say so politely but firmly. Being aggressive is unlikely to help – not least because many receptionists believe that if you are well enough to shout, you are well enough to wait!

- If you want to avoid getting irritated with the system at your surgery, it's worth getting to know it. No system can satisfy everyone, and most surgeries have come up with a compromise to try to deal with conflicting demands. For instance, annoying though it is to have to ring back several times to speak to the doc, it may be because she's been held up seeing patients and doesn't want to interrupt their time with her. Your practice leaflet should have lots of information about opening times, times when the docs take phone calls, the range of staff and facilities, and so on. If the information you want isn't there, it's worth asking the receptionist about it and making a note on your copy of the practice leaflet for future reference.

- An alternative to keeping ringing back is simply to turn up at the surgery to talk to one of the receptionists. We've said it before but we'll say it again – make the receptionist your friend. Receptionists have a tough job – they're constantly trying to juggle the demands of patients (who all want to see someone *now* and all of whom know their problem is more urgent than anyone else's) and GPs, who need things to run smoothly if they are to get everything done. The receptionists will really appreciate it if you are polite and don't hassle them – and if you take the trouble to come in and have a chat when things are relatively quiet, they can give you all sorts of useful tips about how to make the most of the system.

Finally, if you really aren't happy with your surgery or your GP, there's always the option of changing to another practice. You can get details of local surgeries from your Health Authority or Community Health Council (their number should be in the phone book) or the local library. Alternatively, personal reccommendation from a mate should reduce the chance of you ending up at a new practice you rate less than your old one.

How to make the most of seeing your GP

The average GP runs two surgeries a day, each for two or three hours and, contrary to popular belief, does *not* spend the rest of the day playing golf or reading the newspapers. There has always been lots of paperwork as well as visits, phone calls, teaching, and clinics, but these days the time spent in meetings about new medical developments, quality of care, what services patients need, how to save money, and so on is mind-boggling. While this isn't your problem, it may help to explain why it is difficult to get hold of your GP when you want to and why she always seems so stressed when you do see her.

The average GP has about nine minutes per consultation – so if someone takes more than that, everyone who comes after will have to wait that bit longer. It also means you'll want to make the most out of the limited time you've got, which can be really difficult when you're tense or worried. Here, then, are a few tips to try to ensure you leave the surgery feeling you and your GP were on the same wavelength:

- If you've got kids, try to make an appointment when they aren't with you. Even if you think your problem isn't about anything embarrassing, it may turn out to be something you'd rather they didn't pass round their mates in the playground ('So then the doctor asked her to take all her clothes off and got behind the curtain with her and told her it might be a bit uncomfy but she should take some deep breaths . . .'). Also, children can be very distracting when both you and your doc want to concentrate on your problems.

- Think about what she might ask you. If you tell her about a problem, she'll need to find out the facts – so try to get them straight in advance (for instance, if you have a problem with your periods, there's a fair chance she'll want to know the length of your cycle, the date of your last period, and so on).

- Be prepared to be examined. It's astonishing how many women come in with a gynae problem and are surprised when the doc wants to have a look – it's not perversion, just good safe medicine! If you only want to be examined by a woman then don't book in to see a male doc.

- Of course, you do have a right to refuse to be examined. Having said that, your doc is highly unlikely to suggest an examination unless it's needed, and should be very happy to explain exactly why she thinks it's necessary. If that persuades you that you need an exam but you still don't feel comfortable, you do have a right to ask for a chaperone (or to bring your Mum or a friend with you to act as one).

Things not to say to your GP

- 'I don't come very often so I've brought a list.'
- 'I just want some antibiotics.'
- 'I think I've got ME.'
- 'I've got toothache.'
- 'I need an X-ray.'
- 'I've got chronic pain in my solar plexus.'
- 'I just want a letter to see a specialist.'
- 'The TV/radio doc said . . .'/'I cut this out of a newspaper/magazine . . .'
- 'While I'm here, doctor . . .'

- Think about any tests she might want to do. If you have cystitis, for instance, take a urine sample in with you; if you're likely to need a vaginal examination, go in the middle of the month so you don't need to come back after your period, and can get a smear done at the same time if you're due for one. (Of course, if you really don't want to be examined but are embarrassed to say so, you can always pretend you *have* got a period! It doesn't mean you won't need an examination at some point, but it may give you the opportunity to get yourself psyched up for it, or to book an appointment with a doc you feel more comfortable with.) Some blood tests and swabs need to be sent to the lab the same day, so don't make a late evening appointment if you think you might need tests of this sort.

- Show her anything, but don't show her your teeth. Doctors are not dentists. Dentists are dentists. If there's one thing that really sets the average doc's teeth on edge, it's the knowledge that the patient sees her as a more accessible (sees patients at less than a month's notice), cheaper (i.e. free), poor relation to the dentist.

- Saving your problems up and coming in with a long list might seem like the perfect way to get everything out of the way in one go, but you may not get a satisfactory answer to any of them if you do. Your GP won't be able to do all your problems justice in nine minutes, so she may feel pressurized and be forced into a superficial approach. If you want to be able to discuss each problem fully then try to book a double-length appointment (if your surgery allows you to). Alternatively, tell the doc about the problem you think is the most important or give her the list and let her decide what to do with it. The advantage of this is that some medical problems cause symptoms you couldn't know were related but which she might spot straight away. She also might spot that all the symptoms on your list add up to stress/anxiety and focus on that.

- Avoid the 'by the way, doctor' scenario. This is otherwise known as 'while I'm here' or the 'hand on the doorknob' consultation, and is guaranteed to dismay the average GP. Remember those old-fashioned movies about the pubescent male going up to the pharmacy counter for condoms and coming out with two tubes of toothpaste and a dozen bars of soap? Well, that's how 'by the way, doctor' works. For instance, you go in to see the GP (probably one you don't know and certainly don't trust) because you're getting pain when you have sex in certain positions. She looks a bit stern so you test her out by asking about your weight. By the time you've worked out she's human after all and plucked up courage to tell her the real reason you're here, you're at the door on the way out and you've spent nine minutes talking about avoiding chip butties. Now she has to start all over again on the 'real' problem, and is running later and later. You'll get a much better deal from your doctor if you're up front about it – and remember, even if you're embarrassed, she'll have heard it all before.

- Try not to have too many preconceived ideas about what your problem is caused by, or what needs doing about it. It may sometimes feel as if your GP is just a barrier between you and more high-tech medical care, but you're much more likely to be able to have a productive chat about what you want and why if she feels you're interested in what she thinks. Of course your doc is there to make you better if she can – but another important part of her job is protecting you from hospitals if they can be avoided. Many hospital investigations and treatments are unpleasant and some are downright risky. This doesn't

mean she won't refer you for them if you need them – but it does mean that she won't want to put you through them unnecessarily.

- Do tell your GP what you're worried about. Your GP is not a mind-reader, and just because she treated your Aunt Mabel for lung cancer five years ago doesn't mean she'll realize that you think you've got the same when you come in with a cough in the middle of a flu epidemic. While GPs often don't mention the serious things they are ruling out by their questions and examination (for fear of giving you ideas about what terrible conditions you *might* have!), if you tell her what you're worried about, she'll be very happy to explain why she is confident you haven't got it – or why she agrees that you might.

- If you aren't happy with the GP's explanation or suggested treatment, say so. While this gambit doesn't guarantee you'll get what you want, at least you should get a fuller explanation of why she doesn't feel it's appropriate.

Of course, there are still going to be occasions when you leave the surgery wanting to scream. It may be because your GP's having an off day; it may be because in your opinion she's a power-crazy moron and she always will be. It's probably worth letting yourself cool off a bit before you decide what to do about it. Screaming at the receptionists and slamming the door on the way out might make you feel better at the time, but it isn't acceptable behaviour and will colour your relationship with the practice – and you'll feel pretty silly if she turns out to be right.

If you really feel that you have given it your best shot and your GP is still being unreasonable, you can always seek a second opinion – either from another doctor in the surgery or by registering elsewhere. And if all else fails, of course, at least you've got this book to refer to.

Part Two

Diagnose-it-yourself guide

Our flow charts are designed to lead you quickly and pain-lessly to the most likely diagnosis and, in the vast majority of cases, will do just that. However, diseases cannot always be relied upon to follow the usual pattern and may affect you in a different or more worrying way to normal.

Make sure you read the 'How to use this book' section before using the diagnose-it-yourself guide. And remember – the flow charts are an aid. They are not a substitute for your own common sense and judgement. If you have any doubts, particularly when you're in a ⚠ or ⚠ diagnosis area – if your symptoms don't seem to fit a diagnosis or if they seem worse or more serious than the chart suggests – then seek medical advice.

Remember:

⚠ means see your GP sharpish

⚠ means an urgent hospital job

Abdominal pain – one-off

NB. Pregnancy (more than 12 weeks' gestation) causes of abdominal pain are not covered. If you are pregnant and your pain is not obviously caused by a muscle strain or gastroentitis, then seek medical advice.

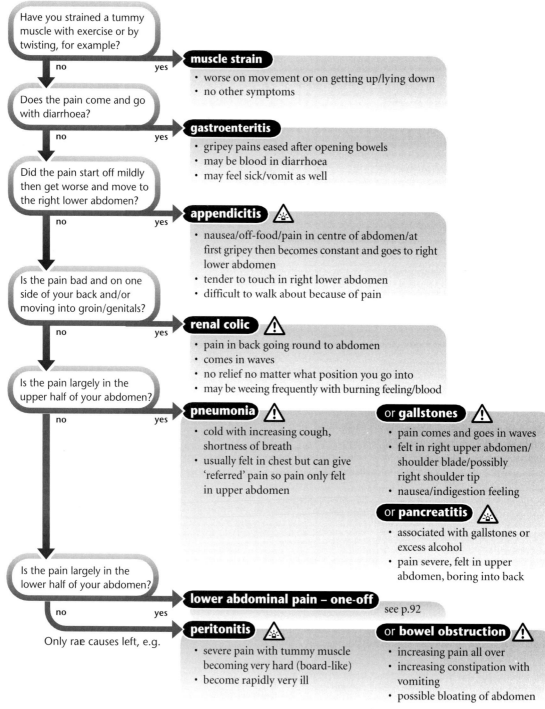

Have you strained a tummy muscle with exercise or by twisting, for example?

muscle strain
- worse on movement or on getting up/lying down
- no other symptoms

Does the pain come and go with diarrhoea?

gastroenteritis
- gripey pains eased after opening bowels
- may be blood in diarrhoea
- may feel sick/vomit as well

Did the pain start off mildly then get worse and move to the right lower abdomen?

appendicitis
- nausea/off-food/pain in centre of abdomen/at first gripey then becomes constant and goes to right lower abdomen
- tender to touch in right lower abdomen
- difficult to walk about because of pain

Is the pain bad and on one side of your back and/or moving into groin/genitals?

renal colic
- pain in back going round to abdomen
- comes in waves
- no relief no matter what position you go into
- may be weeing frequently with burning feeling/blood

Is the pain largely in the upper half of your abdomen?

pneumonia
- cold with increasing cough, shortness of breath
- usually felt in chest but can give 'referred' pain so pain only felt in upper abdomen

or gallstones
- pain comes and goes in waves
- felt in right upper abdomen/shoulder blade/possibly right shoulder tip
- nausea/indigestion feeling

or pancreatitis
- associated with gallstones or excess alcohol
- pain severe, felt in upper abdomen, boring into back

Is the pain largely in the lower half of your abdomen?

lower abdominal pain – one-off
see p.92

Only rae causes left, e.g.

peritonitis
- severe pain with tummy muscle becoming very hard (board-like)
- become rapidly very ill

or bowel obstruction
- increasing pain all over
- increasing constipation with vomiting
- possible bloating of abdomen

 If your abdominal pain is severe, or you feel ill or faint with it, then the actual diagnosis does not matter — it is likely to have a serious cause and you must seek medical attention immediately.

Gastroenteritis A germ in the bowel, usually through something you've eaten – hence the term 'food poisoning'.

Treatment The problem will sort itself out without any treatment, but it can take anything from a few hours to 10 days. All you need to do is drink plenty of clear fluids then start a light diet once any vomiting stops (the diarrhoea usually takes longer). If the diarrhoea is terrible, you may be tempted to get some medicine from the chemist to bung you up, but it's probably better to let the germ simply pass through the system. A hot water bottle and some paracetamol will help ease the gripey pain. Contact your GP if the diarrhoea's showing no signs of settling after 10 days, you're passing a lot of blood, or you've just travelled to somewhere exotic. And if your job involves handling food, don't return to work until the diarrhoea has stopped, and be very careful about hand washing.

Muscle strain A pulled muscle in your abdomen can cause a mild pain.

Treatment Simple – use a painkiller and some heat, take it easy on the sports for a week or two, remember to warm up in future, and it should heal quickly.

Appendicitis The appendix is a useless, worm-like bit of gut. If it becomes inflamed, it swells and causes severe belly ache.

Treatment A hospital job to have it whipped out.

Renal colic This is a stone (usually like a small piece of gravel) in the tube joining the kidney to the bladder. This tube is very thin and muscular, and squeezes hard to push the stone through, causing horrendous pain. Some people have a tendency to keep making stones, and so can get repeated attacks.

Treatment It probably depends who it's quickest to get to – the local hospital or your GP. You'll be in so much pain you won't really care who sees you, you'll just want it sorted out asap. It needs strong painkillers, usually by injection, and a high fluid intake. If your GP does treat you, she may need to send you to hospital anyway if it doesn't quickly

settle down and, especially if it's your first attack, you're likely to need further tests.

Gallstones Stones in the gall bladder, another useless part of the anatomy – a small bag that sits just under the liver. No one knows what causes them, but they can run in families, and they can give repeated attacks of severe stomach ache.

Treatment During an attack of pain (technically, 'biliary colic') you'll need either strong painkillers from your GP or a trip to the hospital. If attacks are frequent and a real nuisance, then the only cure is an operation to remove the gall bladder – and a low fat diet while you're waiting.

Pneumonia This is a severe infection of the lungs. It inflames the lung lining (the pleura), leading to 'pleurisy'. This can cause referred pain in the stomach (pain arising in one place – in this case, the lungs – but felt somewhere else).

Treatment See your GP asap as this needs antibiotics. It can make you quite ill, in which case you'll be sent to hospital.

Pancreatitis and peritonitis Inflammation of the pancreas and the lining of the guts, respectively. Pancreatitis can be caused by a virus, too much alcohol, and gallstones, amongst other things. Peritonitis is usually caused by a hole (a 'perforation') appearing in the bowel courtesy of, for example, appendicitis or a duodenal ulcer.

Treatment Urgent hospital attention is needed for both.

Bowel obstruction If your intestine gets blocked, the muscular walls of your bowel will squeeze to try to push past it. This causes, amongst other symptoms, severe stomach pain. Although it's pretty rare, there are lots of different reasons why your bowel might get blocked – the commonest is probably 'adhesions' (gluey bits which can stick bits of bowel together after previous surgery – such as for appendicitis).

Treatment Your GP will send you to hospital if she thinks you have bowel obstruction.

Abdominal pain – recurrent

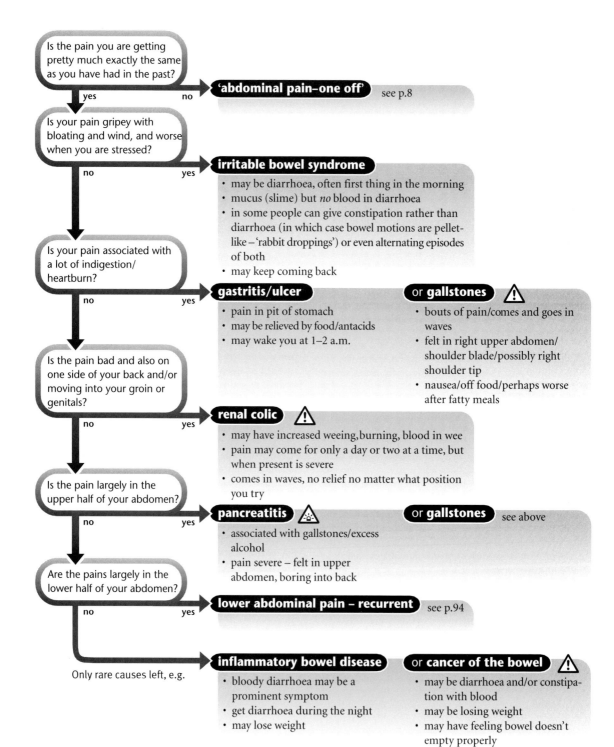

Is the pain you are getting pretty much exactly the same as you have had in the past?

yes → no

'abdominal pain–one off' see p.8

Is your pain gripey with bloating and wind, and worse when you are stressed?

no / yes →

irritable bowel syndrome
- may be diarrhoea, often first thing in the morning
- mucus (slime) but *no* blood in diarrhoea
- in some people can give constipation rather than diarrhoea (in which case bowel motions are pellet-like – 'rabbit droppings') or even alternating episodes of both
- may keep coming back

Is your pain associated with a lot of indigestion/heartburn?

no / yes →

gastritis/ulcer
- pain in pit of stomach
- may be relieved by food/antacids
- may wake you at 1–2 a.m.

or gallstones ⚠
- bouts of pain/comes and goes in waves
- felt in right upper abdomen/shoulder blade/possibly right shoulder tip
- nausea/off food/perhaps worse after fatty meals

Is the pain bad and also on one side of your back and/or moving into your groin or genitals?

no / yes →

renal colic ⚠
- may have increased weeing, burning, blood in wee
- pain may come for only a day or two at a time, but when present is severe
- comes in waves, no relief no matter what position you try

Is the pain largely in the upper half of your abdomen?

no / yes →

pancreatitis ⚠

or gallstones see above
- associated with gallstones/excess alcohol
- pain severe – felt in upper abdomen, boring into back

Are the pains largely in the lower half of your abdomen?

no / yes →

lower abdominal pain – recurrent see p.94

Only rare causes left, e.g. →

inflammatory bowel disease
- bloody diarrhoea may be a prominent symptom
- get diarrhoea during the night
- may lose weight

or cancer of the bowel ⚠
- may be diarrhoea and/or constipation with blood
- may be losing weight
- may have feeling bowel doesn't empty properly

Irritable bowel syndrome (IBS) The bowel is simply a long muscular tube. When 'irritable', it squeezes too much, too little, or in an uncoordinated way, resulting in the typical symptoms of IBS.

Treatment No one's absolutely sure what causes this problem but it's very common and, though troublesome, is harmless. Avoid any particular foods which you find aggravate it, increase your fibre if you get a lot of constipation, but decrease it if bloating is a big problem. It's worth cutting down on cigarettes, alcohol, and caffeine (in coffee, tea, and cola) too. Physical exercise, and relaxation exercises to reduce stress, may help. If the pain is very distressing then antispasmodic treatment, available from the chemist, may give some relief. And if it's getting really bad, or it's getting you down, discuss the problem with your GP, who may try other treatments – but bear in mind that there's no magic answer.

Gastritis/ulcer The stomach produces acid to help digest the food. But sometimes the acid can inflame the stomach lining – 'gastritis' – causing an indigestion-type pain. Occasionally, the acid burns a small crater in the lining of the duodenum, the tube which carries food away from the stomach – this is a duodenal ulcer. This type of problem sometimes runs in families and can be caused, or aggravated, by alcohol, acidic medication (such as aspirin or ibuprofen), and a poor diet. A gastric ulcer is the same thing, but in the stomach – and it usually occurs in an older age group (the over 40s, whereas a duodenal ulcer tends to affect those aged between 20 and 50).

Treatment For mild acid problems, look at your diet and lifestyle. Avoid spicy foods, eat regularly, and cut down on cigarettes and alcohol. Also, steer clear of some acidic over-the-counter painkillers like aspirin and ibuprofen; paracetamol is OK. The chemist will be able to give you an antacid which should help. If the problem doesn't settle, or your symptoms point to an ulcer, see your GP – she can prescribe effective treatments to cut down the acid, and in some cases, treatments which might cure the problem once and for all.

Renal colic This is explained in the 'Abdominal pain – one off' section (p. 8). Some people tend to keep developing stones and so can suffer repeated attacks of renal colic.

Treatment The treatment of an attack is discussed in the 'Abdominal pain – one-off' section (p. 8). If you get repeated attacks, your GP will have you checked out to see if there's any reason why you keep developing stones. It's important to drink plenty, and you may be given dietary advice, or some medication, to cut down the chances of further problems.

Gallstones This is explained in the 'Abdominal pain – one-off' section (p. 8). The pain may come back again, especially after fatty meals, until the problem is sorted out once and for all.

Treatment See the 'Abdominal pain – one-off' section (p. 8). If attacks are frequent and a real nuisance, then the only cure is an operation to remove the gall bladder.

Pancreatitis This is an inflamed pancreas – a bit of your innards which sits deep in the pit of your stomach and helps digest your food. It usually gets inflamed either because of gallstones or too much alcohol.

Treatment You shouldn't be in much doubt about what to do during an attack – the pain is bad and you'll feel pretty ill, so hospital is the obvious option. Preventing repeated attacks depends on the cause and might involve you having your gallstones sorted out or cutting out the alcohol.

Other medical problems Very occasionally, repeated attacks of stomach ache are caused by some other problem, such as a swollen kidney, inflammatory bowel disease (see the 'Diarrhoea' section, p. 50), side-effects of medication, or bowel cancer (rare in the under 50s).

Treatment See your GP if you think you might have a problem of this sort – she will arrange any necessary tests.

Abdominal swelling or bloating

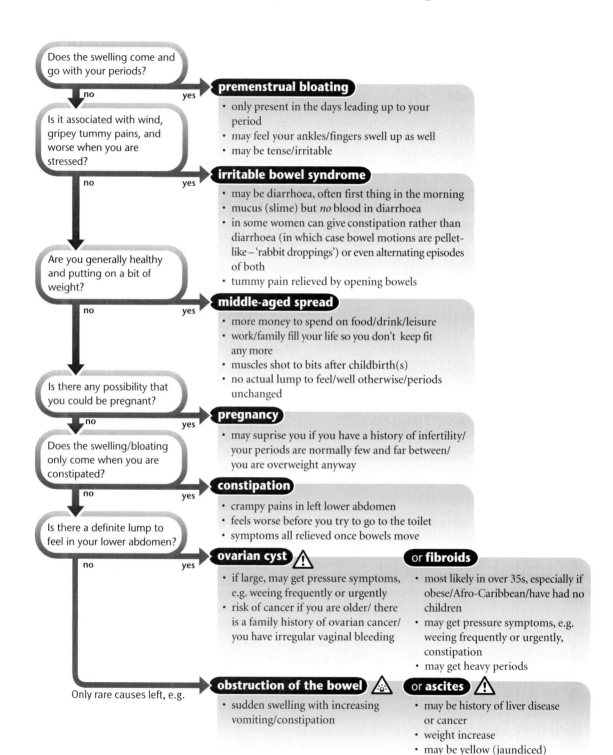

Does the swelling come and go with your periods? — yes →

premenstrual bloating
- only present in the days leading up to your period
- may feel your ankles/fingers swell up as well
- may be tense/irritable

Is it associated with wind, gripey tummy pains, and worse when you are stressed? — yes →

irritable bowel syndrome
- may be diarrhoea, often first thing in the morning
- mucus (slime) but *no* blood in diarrhoea
- in some women can give constipation rather than diarrhoea (in which case bowel motions are pellet-like – 'rabbit droppings') or even alternating episodes of both
- tummy pain relieved by opening bowels

Are you generally healthy and putting on a bit of weight? — yes →

middle-aged spread
- more money to spend on food/drink/leisure
- work/family fill your life so you don't keep fit any more
- muscles shot to bits after childbirth(s)
- no actual lump to feel/well otherwise/periods unchanged

Is there any possibility that you could be pregnant? — yes →

pregnancy
- may suprise you if you have a history of infertility/ your periods are normally few and far between/ you are overweight anyway

Does the swelling/bloating only come when you are constipated? — yes →

constipation
- crampy pains in left lower abdomen
- feels worse before you try to go to the toilet
- symptoms all relieved once bowels move

Is there a definite lump to feel in your lower abdomen? — yes →

ovarian cyst ⚠
- if large, may get pressure symptoms, e.g. weeing frequently or urgently
- risk of cancer if you are older/ there is a family history of ovarian cancer/ you have irregular vaginal bleeding

or fibroids
- most likely in over 35s, especially if obese/Afro-Caribbean/have had no children
- may get pressure symptoms, e.g. weeing frequently or urgently, constipation
- may get heavy periods

Only rare causes left, e.g.

obstruction of the bowel ⚠
- sudden swelling with increasing vomiting/constipation

or ascites ⚠
- may be history of liver disease or cancer
- weight increase
- may be yellow (jaundiced)

Abdominal swelling or bloating

Premenstrual bloating Actual swelling, or a bloated feeling, may occur in the days leading up to your period – either on its own or as a part of 'premenstrual syndrome'. This is commonly known as 'fluid retention', though whether the symptoms are actually caused by the body retaining fluid isn't clear.

Treatment There's no magic solution for this problem. Although diuretics ('water tablets') have been tried, they probably don't really help in the long run and they can have side-effects – so most doctors don't prescribe them these days. You're more likely to ease the problem with self-help measures such as a healthy diet, regular exercise, and relaxation therapy. If your bloating is only one part of premenstrual syndrome, check out the treatments suggested in the relevant part of the 'Feeling tense' section (p. 64).

Irritable bowel syndrome (IBS) Bloating is a common symptom experienced by irritable bowel sufferers. For further details of this problem, see the 'Abdominal pain – recurrent' section (p. 10).

Treatment It may be worth cutting down on fizzy drinks and fibre – a high fibre diet is traditionally recommended for IBS but it can actually make the bloating worse, especially in the short term. For further advice about treating irritable bowel, see the 'Abdominal pain – recurrent' section (p. 10).

'Middle-aged spread' A common cause for a mild and gradual swelling of the abdomen is simply excess fat. This is explained further, together with advice on slimming down, in the 'Weight gain' section (p. 162).

Pregnancy You don't need a medical qualification to realize that pregnancy will cause abdominal swelling, usually noticed from about 16 weeks onwards. But it's very unlikely that the swelling will bring the pregnancy to your attention – unless you've not noticed, or chosen to ignore, the nausea, breast tenderness, lack of periods, and frequent trips to the loo.

Constipation This is explained in the 'Abnormal bowel motions' section (p. 14). Severe constipation may make your tummy swell or, more likely, make you feel very bloated.

Treatment This is explained in the 'Abnormal bowel motions' section (p. 14).

Ovarian cyst This is a fluid-filled swelling on your ovary. It can get very large – up to the size of a basketball. Usually these cysts are 'harmless', apart from the discomfort they cause, but occasionally they can be caused by a cancer of the ovary. Cancer is far less likely if you have been on the contraceptive pill and/or had children, but it's more of a possibility if there is a history of ovarian cancer in your family.

Treatment Your GP will refer you to a gynaecologist to have the ovarian cyst removed – this will make you more comfortable and means that the swelling can be analysed for any signs of cancer.

Fibroids These are benign lumps in the muscle wall of the womb. They can sometimes grow large enough to cause a swelling in the lower part of your abdomen.

Treatment This is explained in the 'Heavy periods' section (p.72).

Medical rarities Very unusual problems such as obstruction of the bowel or a large accumulation of fluid inside your abdomen ('ascites' – usually caused by a serious illness) can cause swelling.

Treatment It's highly unlikely that you'll suffer any of these problems – and if you do, you'll have lots of other symptoms to alert you that something is seriously wrong. If your GP is concerned that you might have one of these rarities, she'll refer you to a specialist.

Abnormal bowel motions

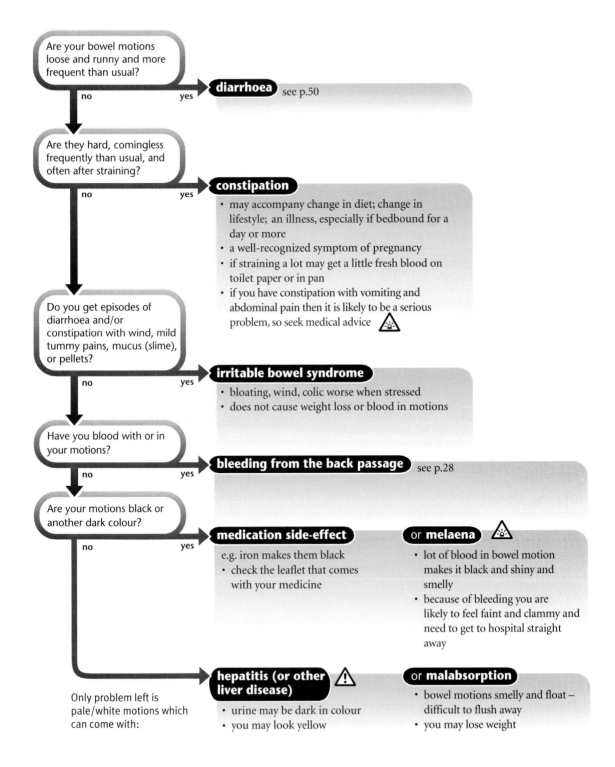

Are your bowel motions loose and runny and more frequent than usual?

no / yes

diarrhoea see p.50

Are they hard, comingless frequently than usual, and often after straining?

no / yes

constipation
- may accompany change in diet; change in lifestyle; an illness, especially if bedbound for a day or more
- a well-recognized symptom of pregnancy
- if straining a lot may get a little fresh blood on toilet paper or in pan
- if you have constipation with vomiting and abdominal pain then it is likely to be a serious problem, so seek medical advice

Do you get episodes of diarrhoea and/or constipation with wind, mild tummy pains, mucus (slime), or pellets?

no / yes

irritable bowel syndrome
- bloating, wind, colic worse when stressed
- does not cause weight loss or blood in motions

Have you blood with or in your motions?

no / yes

bleeding from the back passage see p.28

Are your motions black or another dark colour?

no / yes

medication side-effect
e.g. iron makes them black
- check the leaflet that comes with your medicine

or melaena
- lot of blood in bowel motion makes it black and shiny and smelly
- because of bleeding you are likely to feel faint and clammy and need to get to hospital straight away

Only problem left is pale/white motions which can come with:

hepatitis (or other liver disease)
- urine may be dark in colour
- you may look yellow

or malabsorption
- bowel motions smelly and float – difficult to flush away
- you may lose weight

Abnormal bowel motions

Diarrhoea See the 'Diarrhoea' section, (p. 50).

Constipation This means difficulty in opening your bowels – in other words, having to strain a lot when you go. A hectic lifestyle, a poor diet, and a lack of exercise are the usual causes. Pregnancy (especially if you're taking iron tablets) can also bung you up. Some medications (such as antidepressants and painkillers containing codeine) can cause constipation, as can some illicit drugs (like heroin). A vicious cycle can develop: constipation might cause an anal fissure (see the 'Pain in the bottom' section p. 112) which, in turn, makes you unwilling to go, causing further constipation. Rarely, constipation coming on suddenly over a day or two can be the result of a blockage in your bowel ('intestinal obstruction'). This can be caused by a number of things and also results in severe stomach ache and swelling, and vomiting.

Treatment Increase your fibre intake. This means more fruit, vegetables, and bran. Also, take more exercise, as this helps stimulate the bowels. Try to make use of the early morning urge to go, which usually comes on about half an hour after eating breakfast – so give yourself an extra 10 minutes in the morning to sit on the loo. If you think that some medication you're taking may be causing the problem, have a word with your chemist or GP, as you may be able to stop it or try an alternative. And while you're in the chemist's, you might try a laxative such as senna tablets: this will help get you going, though it's best used only for a short time while you're sorting out your diet and some exercise. If you get a real pain in the bottom when you try to go, you've probably got an anal fissure – see the 'Pain in the bottom' section (p. 112) for advice on how to treat this. Constipation caused by intestinal obstruction needs urgent medical treatment – go to casualty.

Irritable bowel syndrome See the 'Diarrhoea' (p. 50) and 'Abdominal pain' (p. 8) sections for details about this condition and how it's treated. If you suffer from irritable bowel syndrome, you can get constipation or diarrhoea, or both – and you may pass mucus and stuff that looks like rabbit droppings. Constipation, in particular, can get worse premenstrually.

Bleeding from the back passage See the 'Bleeding from the back passage' section (p. 28).

Melaena This is the passage of jet-black, tarry motions which usually smell disgusting. It is caused by blood which has been altered as it has passed through the bowel, and it means you're bleeding somewhere in your gut – from a duodenal ulcer, for example.

Treatment You need urgent medical attention, so get to casualty asap.

Medication side-effect Some medicines can change the colour of your motions. For example, iron turns them black.

Treatment Check the leaflet in the treatment pack or speak to the chemist to see if your coloured motions are a recognized side-effect of the treatment you're taking. If you're not sure, and your problem is black motions, speak to your GP to make sure it's not melaena (see above).

Hepatitis (or other similar problem) Hepatitis is inflammation of the liver, usually caused by a virus. Some types (such as hepatitis A) are caught just like tummy bugs; more serious sorts (like hepatitis B and C) are usually passed on sexually or through infected blood (e.g. sharing needles if you inject drugs). Swelling in the liver stops a pigment getting through to your bowels, so you end up with pale motions, although you're likely to notice other symptoms too – such as turning yellow (jaundice). A number of other problems can have the same effect, including some medications and gallstones.

Treatment See your GP. She'll need to run some tests to work out exactly what the problem is, and she may need to refer you to a specialist.

Malabsorption This is explained in the 'Diarrhoea' section (p. 50). Some types of malabsorption cause pale, floating motions that can be hard to flush away.

Abnormal or irregular vaginal bleeding

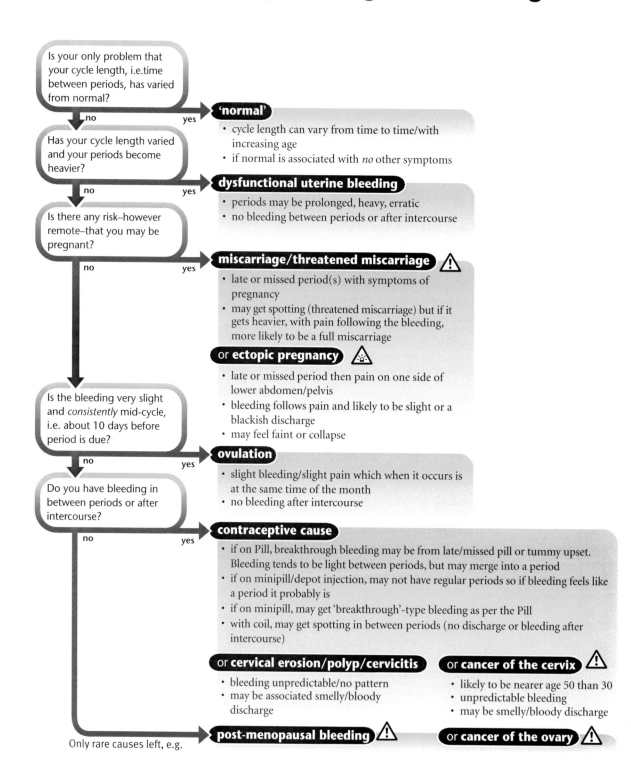

Is your only problem that your cycle length, i.e.time between periods, has varied from normal?

no → yes

'normal'
- cycle length can vary from time to time/with increasing age
- if normal is associated with *no* other symptoms

Has your cycle length varied and your periods become heavier?

no → yes

dysfunctional uterine bleeding
- periods may be prolonged, heavy, erratic
- no bleeding between periods or after intercourse

Is there any risk–however remote–that you may be pregnant?

no → yes

miscarriage/threatened miscarriage ⚠
- late or missed period(s) with symptoms of pregnancy
- may get spotting (threatened miscarriage) but if it gets heavier, with pain following the bleeding, more likely to be a full miscarriage

or ectopic pregnancy ⚠
- late or missed period then pain on one side of lower abdomen/pelvis
- bleeding follows pain and likely to be slight or a blackish discharge
- may feel faint or collapse

Is the bleeding very slight and *consistently* mid-cycle, i.e. about 10 days before period is due?

no → yes

ovulation
- slight bleeding/slight pain which when it occurs is at the same time of the month
- no bleeding after intercourse

Do you have bleeding in between periods or after intercourse?

no → yes

contraceptive cause
- if on Pill, breakthrough bleeding may be from late/missed pill or tummy upset. Bleeding tends to be light between periods, but may merge into a period
- if on minipill/depot injection, may not have regular periods so if bleeding feels like a period it probably is
- if on minipill, may get 'breakthrough'-type bleeding as per the Pill
- with coil, may get spotting in between periods (no discharge or bleeding after intercourse)

or cervical erosion/polyp/cervicitis
- bleeding unpredictable/no pattern
- may be associated smelly/bloody discharge

or cancer of the cervix ⚠
- likely to be nearer age 50 than 30
- unpredictable bleeding
- may be smelly/bloody discharge

Only rare causes left, e.g.

post-menopausal bleeding ⚠

or cancer of the ovary ⚠

'Normal' Many human characteristics vary: height, weight, appetite, complexion, etc. And so it is with the menstrual cycle – while a 28-day gap between periods is common, it's certainly not the only normal pattern of bleeding. Many women have a shorter or longer cycle or vary from one to the other. This is especially common in the first year or two that periods start and also around the time of the menopause. You don't need to consult your doctor unless you get bleeding in between the periods, bleeding after intercourse, or the periods become unusually heavy.

Contraceptive cause Bleeding which happens while you're on the Pill is quite common and is known as 'breakthrough bleeding'. This may happen for no particular reason, particularly in the first few months of taking the Pill, or there may be a specific cause – for example, a tummy upset, a course of antibiotics, or a missed pill, all of which can cause a drop in hormones enough to result in temporary breakthrough bleeding. Other forms of contraception can cause problems too: the coil can cause spotting in between periods (especially in the first few months of using a hormone-releasing coil), and the minipill and contraceptive injections can lead to irregular periods.

Treatment If you've recently started the Pill, or you think there is a clear cause for your breakthrough bleeding (see above), it's worth waiting and seeing as the problem will usually settle down. If it persists, see your GP as you may need a change of pill or a different type of family planning, and she'll want to check that there's no other cause for the symptom. With the other types of contraception mentioned above, it's worth discussing the situation with your GP. Once you know it's your contraception causing the problem, you have the choice of continuing as you are and putting up with it, or changing to another method of family planning.

Miscarriage/threatened miscarriage It's very common to suffer some spotting early in pregnancy (usually before 12 weeks' gestation) – this is a 'threatened miscarriage'. An actual miscarriage occurs when the bleeding gets much heavier, with pain, and the fetus (the early developing baby) is lost. Sadly, this is quite common: around one in six pregnancies end in a miscarriage, usually because there was a problem with the baby.

Treatment There's no treatment that can prevent a 'threatened' from developing into a proper miscarriage. Bed rest makes no difference and, thankfully, the majority settle down to a normal pregnancy. Some doctors arrange a scan to make sure that all is well, so it's worth discussing the problem with your GP if the spotting goes on for more than a day or two. If it does develop into a proper miscarriage, the bleeding can get quite heavy, so you need to go straight to hospital. As miscarriage is so common, doctors don't routinely do tests to find out why it's happened unless you've been unlucky enough to have three or more in a row.

Cervical erosion/polyp/cervicitis Erosions (which are like grazes of the cervix and often occur for no obvious reason) and polyps (small gristly lumps) can cause bleeding in between periods or after sex. So too can 'cervicitis', which is an infection of the cervix, often caused by a particular germ known as 'chlamydia', which is passed on through sex.

Treatment As you cannot tell whether these symptoms are being caused by a more serious problem – like cancer of the cervix, for example – it's important to get checked out by your GP. Polyps and erosions, if troublesome, are easily treated with very minor surgery – your GP will, if necessary, refer you to a gynaecologist. If you have a chlamydia infection, your GP will probably send you to a local clinic for genito-urinary medicine, where you can be treated and checked for other sexually transmitted infections. Try to persuade your partner to go too, so he can also be checked out.

Dysfunctional uterine bleeding See 'Heavy periods' (p. 72). It may also cause prolonged and erratic periods.

Ovulation It's quite common for women to lose a small amount of blood in mid-cycle, when the egg is released.

Treatment This is quite normal and needs no checking out or treatment, so long as there's no real change in the pattern.

Ectopic pregnancy This is a pregnancy which develops in the Fallopian tube (which joins the womb to the ovary) rather than in the womb. It can cause slight spotting or a blackish discharge. See the 'Lower abdominal pain – one-off' section (p. 92).

Cancer of the cervix Cancer of the neck of the womb can cause irregular bleeding, bleeding after sex, or a blood-stained discharge. While it's likely that these symptoms will be caused by the more harmless problems outlined above, it's important to get checked out by your GP. Remember that you should do this even if a recent smear was normal – cancers can sometimes develop regardless of smear test results.

Treatment If your GP is worried you might have this type of problem, she'll refer you urgently to a gynaecologist for a colposcopy – a detailed look at the cervix through a type of telescope – and appropriate treatment.

Other rare problems Other rare problems, including different types of cancer, can cause irregular bleeding.

Treatment See your GP to get the symptoms checked out.

Absent periods

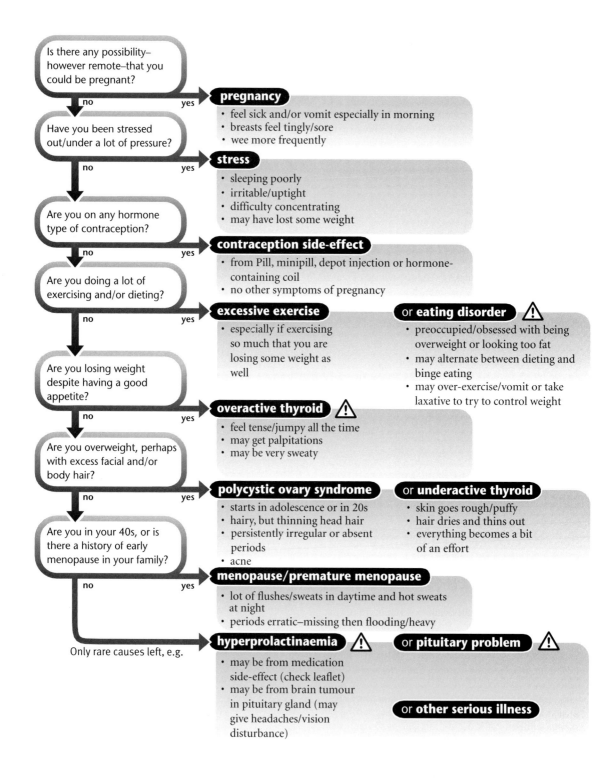

Is there any possibility–
however remote–that you
could be pregnant?

no   yes

pregnancy
- feel sick and/or vomit especially in morning
- breasts feel tingly/sore
- wee more frequently

Have you been stressed
out/under a lot of pressure?

no   yes

stress
- sleeping poorly
- irritable/uptight
- difficulty concentrating
- may have lost some weight

Are you on any hormone
type of contraception?

no   yes

contraception side-effect
- from Pill, minipill, depot injection or hormone-containing coil
- no other symptoms of pregnancy

Are you doing a lot of
exercising and/or dieting?

no   yes

excessive exercise
- especially if exercising so much that you are losing some weight as well

or eating disorder
- preoccupied/obsessed with being overweight or looking too fat
- may alternate between dieting and binge eating
- may over-exercise/vomit or take laxative to try to control weight

Are you losing weight
despite having a good
appetite?

no   yes

overactive thyroid
- feel tense/jumpy all the time
- may get palpitations
- may be very sweaty

Are you overweight, perhaps
with excess facial and/or
body hair?

no   yes

polycystic ovary syndrome
- starts in adolescence or in 20s
- hairy, but thinning head hair
- persistently irregular or absent periods
- acne

or underactive thyroid
- skin goes rough/puffy
- hair dries and thins out
- everything becomes a bit of an effort

Are you in your 40s, or is
there a history of early
menopause in your family?

no   yes

menopause/premature menopause
- lot of flushes/sweats in daytime and hot sweats at night
- periods erratic–missing then flooding/heavy

Only rare causes left, e.g.

hyperprolactinaemia
- may be from medication side-effect (check leaflet)
- may be from brain tumour in pituitary gland (may give headaches/vision disturbance)

or pituitary problem

or other serious illness

Pregnancy This is the first thing many women consider when they miss a period or two – and quite right too, as it's a very likely cause. Never assume you're not pregnant just because you've been using contraception regularly – accidents do happen!

Treatment Confirm this is the cause by getting a pregnancy test from the chemist. These are usually very reliable. Next, see your GP to discuss the result.

Stress Being stressed out can affect your hormones – especially if you've lost weight too – resulting in your periods packing up. Stress from being worried that you might be pregnant may affect your periods too.

Treatment See the 'Lifestyle/stress' part of the 'Feeling tense' section (p. 64) and eat well to try to regain any weight you've lost.

Contraception side-effect Quite a few women on the Pill or Mini-pill find that their periods stop. This does not mean that the Pill isn't working, or that you're 'retaining' the blood of your period. It simply means that the Pill you're on is not building up any lining on your womb, so there is none to be shed each month. About half of women who use the contraception injection, and many who use a coil which releases the hormone progestogen, also find that their periods stop.

Treatment So long as you're sure there's no chance you're pregnant (which is only likely to worry you when you first notice your lack of periods), there's no need for any treatment – though if this is the first period you have missed you might feel happier doing a pregnancy test, as pregnancy is an outside possibility, especially if you have missed a Pill (or Pills). Not having periods with these types of contraception is totally harmless. If you're not happy with the situation, and would rather see a regular monthly cycle, then you'll need to change your brand of Pill or your method of contraception, so see your GP.

Excessive exercise The type of exercise taken by serious athletes and ballet dancers can – especially if linked with weight loss – cause hormone changes which will stop the periods.

Treatment Ease up on the training, if possible, and get back to your normal weight.

Polycystic ovary syndrome In this condition, many small cysts develop on your ovaries. They produce a hormone called 'testosterone', resulting in a hormone imbalance which makes your periods stop and can cause other problems such as excessive hair growth.

Treatment Many women with troublesome polycystic ovary syndrome are overweight. A healthy diet resulting in weight loss may be all the treatment that's needed. If you don't succeed, or this doesn't bring the periods back on its own, then it's worth seeing your GP. Your doctor's approach will depend mainly on whether or not you're wanting to fall pregnant. If you are, then you may need treatment to help stimulate your ovaries, which may mean being referred to a gynaecologist. If not, then a hormone treatment (such as the contraceptive pill) can be used to restart your menstrual cycle. The treatment of excess hair in polycystic ovary syndrome is discussed in the 'Excessive hair' section (p. 60).

Eating disorder The weight loss caused by the eating disorder anorexia nervosa causes hormone changes which stop the normal menstrual cycle. Further details, and an outline of treatment, are provided in the 'Weight loss' section (p. 164). Many women go through phases of faddy dieting which can affect their periods. This is usually temporary but, if severe and prolonged, can progress to anorexia nervosa.

Menopause/premature menopause This is discussed in the 'Flushing' section (p. 66).

Hyperprolactinaemia Prolactin is a hormone normally produced in small amounts by the 'pituitary gland' in the brain. Prolactin levels rise during pregnancy as this hormone is responsible for breast growth and milk development. Some illnesses (such as growths on the pituitary) and some drugs (especially treatments for psychiatric conditions) can lead to very high levels of prolactin. This is known as 'hyperprolactinaemia', and the hormone imbalance it causes can stop the periods.

Treatment If the problem is a side-effect of drugs, then it may be best to ignore it or to consider a change in treatment – discuss the situation with your GP. A growth on the pituitary will need specialist treatment, so your GP will refer you to a hospital consultant.

Thyroid problems An under- or overactive thyroid gland can stop the normal menstrual cycle. These problems are discussed, and their treatments outlined, in the 'Weight gain' (p. 162) and 'Excess sweating' (p. 58) sections respectively.

Rare problems A few rarities, such as pituitary disorders and other severe illnesses, can stop your periods.

Treatment See your GP if you're concerned, though any rare serious problem will be likely to show itself with various other symptoms unrelated to your menstrual cycle.

Ankle swelling

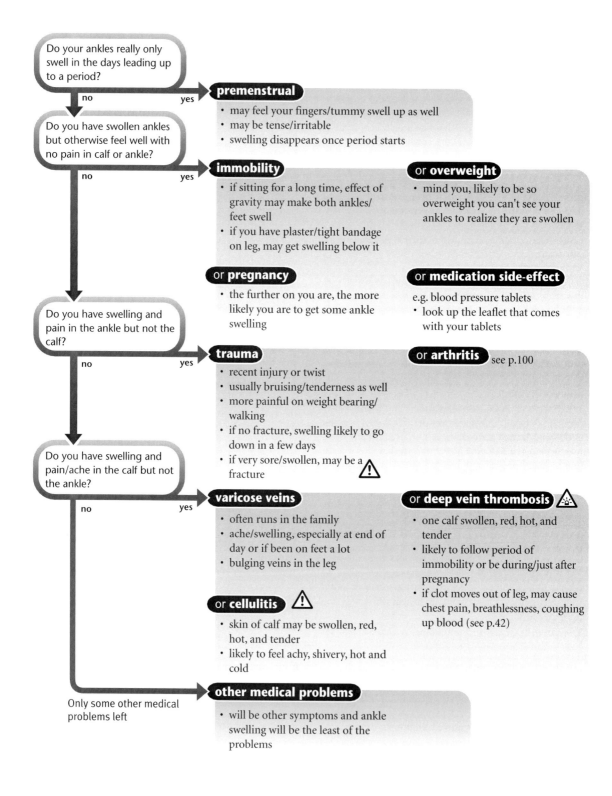

Do your ankles really only swell in the days leading up to a period?
— no → / yes →

premenstrual
- may feel your fingers/tummy swell up as well
- may be tense/irritable
- swelling disappears once period starts

Do you have swollen ankles but otherwise feel well with no pain in calf or ankle?
— no → / yes →

immobility
- if sitting for a long time, effect of gravity may make both ankles/ feet swell
- if you have plaster/tight bandage on leg, may get swelling below it

or overweight
- mind you, likely to be so overweight you can't see your ankles to realize they are swollen

or pregnancy
- the further on you are, the more likely you are to get some ankle swelling

or medication side-effect
e.g. blood pressure tablets
- look up the leaflet that comes with your tablets

Do you have swelling and pain in the ankle but not the calf?
— no → / yes →

trauma
- recent injury or twist
- usually bruising/tenderness as well
- more painful on weight bearing/ walking
- if no fracture, swelling likely to go down in a few days
- if very sore/swollen, may be a fracture ⚠

or arthritis see p.100

Do you have swelling and pain/ache in the calf but not the ankle?
— no → / yes →

varicose veins
- often runs in the family
- ache/swelling, especially at end of day or if been on feet a lot
- bulging veins in the leg

or deep vein thrombosis ⚠
- one calf swollen, red, hot, and tender
- likely to follow period of immobility or be during/just after pregnancy
- if clot moves out of leg, may cause chest pain, breathlessness, coughing up blood (see p.42)

or cellulitis ⚠
- skin of calf may be swollen, red, hot, and tender
- likely to feel achy, shivery, hot and cold

Only some other medical problems left

other medical problems
- will be other symptoms and ankle swelling will be the least of the problems

Trauma Going over on your ankle can cause a sprain or fracture. A sprain means that the ligament (the piece of gristle) attaching the outer part of your ankle to your foot is partially torn. In a fracture, part of the ankle is broken or pulled off by the ligament. Both cause swelling as fluid escapes into the injured joint.

Treatment If the ankle is very painful or tender, there is severe swelling, or you can't take your own weight, you need to go to casualty as you may have a fracture. A sprain needs rest for a couple of days (preferably elevated on a stool), ice-packs, and a firm bandage. Painkillers or anti-inflammatory tablets (available over the counter) will relieve the pain. Then you need to get gently moving on your ankle. Some sprains take months to heal and continue to ache and swell for a while whenever you exercise. Physiotherapy and strapping may help. When the ankle feels better and you're more confident on it, you may find that running along (not up and down) a gentle slope like a beach or the camber of a road helps strengthen the joint.

Immobility If you're unable to move about much – perhaps because you're physically handicapped in some way, recovering from an injury, or on a long flight – your ankles may swell, particularly as the day goes on. This is because, as you walk, your calf muscles help your circulation by pumping the blood back up to your heart. When you're immobile, this doesn't happen, so the blood tends to pool in your legs, causing swelling.

Treatment Depending on the circumstances, there may be little you can do about this. If the swelling bothers you, keep your legs up on a stool as much as possible, and pump your calf muscles from time to time. Compression stockings – available from the chemist – can help too.

Overweight The excess fat presses on your blood vessels in the same way that a baby does – see 'Pregnancy' below.

Treatment If you're fat enough to be getting swollen ankles, you have a serious weight problem and need to shed a good few pounds. For further details, see the 'Weight gain' section (p. 162).

Pregnancy Your baby squashes the blood vessels which bring the blood back from your legs. As a result, they leak fluid, causing swollen ankles. Very rarely, swelling of the ankles (and sometimes, swelling elsewhere, such as the face and hands) can be a sign of pre-eclampsia – a complication of pregnancy in which the blood pressure goes up, and which can be dangerous for you and the baby.

Treatment Mild swelling in both ankles during pregnancy is quite normal and harmless, and so needs no treatment. Any suspicion of the much rarer pre-eclampsia requires an urgent (same day) assessment by your GP or midwife – take a specimen of urine with you to be tested.

Premenstrual Ankle swelling can be a part of pre-menstrual bloating – see the 'Abdominal swelling or bloating' section (p. 12) for further details.

Varicose veins These are bendy, bloated blood vessels which draw the blood back from your legs and point it in the direction of your heart. They tend to leak fluid, and this pools around the ankles. There are a number of reasons why your veins might become 'varicose' including having children, being overweight, or suffering a previous 'deep vein thrombosis' (see below). Often, they simply run in the family.

Treatment Slim down if you're overweight. Take regular exercise and try wearing compression stockings if the swelling really bothers you. Surgery can be used for varicose veins but they tend to come again, especially in future pregnancies – discuss the situation with your GP if they're a real nuisance.

Arthritis Various types of arthritis can affect the ankles, causing painful swelling – see the 'Multiple joint pains' section (p. 100) for further details.

Medication side-effect Some prescribed treatments, such as blood pressure pills and anti-inflammatory drugs, can cause ankle swelling as a side-effect.

Treatment Look at the leaflet that comes in the pack. If it mentions swollen ankles as a possible side-effect, and the problem bothers you, discuss the situation with your GP.

Deep vein thrombosis This is explained, and the treatment outlined, in the 'Calf pain' section (p. 42).

Cellulitis This means an infection of the skin. The lower leg is a favourite site for germs getting into the skin, and the infection will result in swelling.

Treatment See your GP – this needs antibiotics.

Some other medical problems A few small-print but serious diseases can make you retain fluid, leading to ankle swelling. These include kidney, liver, and bowel disease and anaemia.

Treatment Ankle swelling usually happens pretty late on in any of these diseases, so it's very unlikely that they'll come to light as a result of this symptom. If you're concerned, speak to your GP.

Arm pain

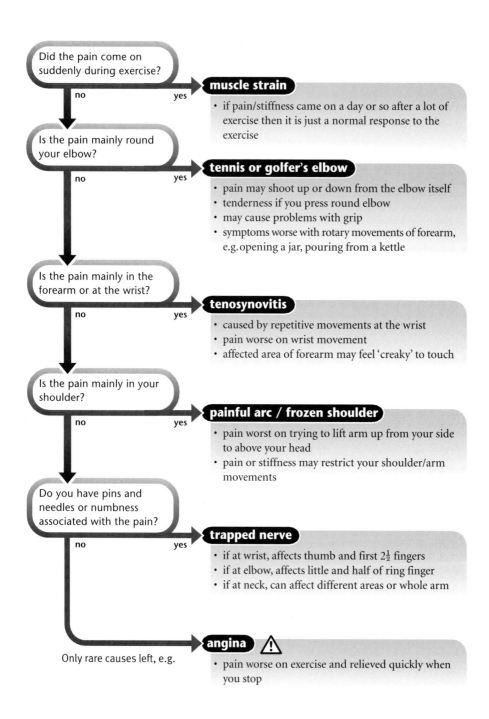

Did the pain come on suddenly during exercise?

no → yes →

muscle strain
- if pain/stiffness came on a day or so after a lot of exercise then it is just a normal response to the exercise

Is the pain mainly round your elbow?

no → yes →

tennis or golfer's elbow
- pain may shoot up or down from the elbow itself
- tenderness if you press round elbow
- may cause problems with grip
- symptoms worse with rotary movements of forearm, e.g. opening a jar, pouring from a kettle

Is the pain mainly in the forearm or at the wrist?

no → yes →

tenosynovitis
- caused by repetitive movements at the wrist
- pain worse on wrist movement
- affected area of forearm may feel 'creaky' to touch

Is the pain mainly in your shoulder?

no → yes →

painful arc / frozen shoulder
- pain worst on trying to lift arm up from your side to above your head
- pain or stiffness may restrict your shoulder/arm movements

Do you have pins and needles or numbness associated with the pain?

no → yes →

trapped nerve
- if at wrist, affects thumb and first $2\frac{1}{2}$ fingers
- if at elbow, affects little and half of ring finger
- if at neck, can affect different areas or whole arm

Only rare causes left, e.g.

angina
- pain worse on exercise and relieved quickly when you stop

Remember: ⚠ means see your GP sharpish; ⚠ means an urgent hospital job

Muscle strain The arm contains a variety of muscles, any of which are easily strained (in other words, over-stretched or partially torn) by, for example, lifting a heavy weight or injuring yourself during sport.

Treatment A mild strain doesn't need any treatment at all and will heal itself in a day or two. A more severe strain needs rest for a few days, an ice-pack (such as a bag of frozen peas wrapped in a towel) on the injured part, and some painkillers or anti-inflammatories (such as ibuprofen, which is available over the counter).

Tennis and golfer's elbow A variety of muscles help you to move your hand at the wrist. Many of these are attached to the elbow – those which pull your hand up are connected to the outer side of the elbow and those which push it down, to the inner side. The areas where these muscles attach can become inflamed – often for no reason, but sometimes through an injury or repeated use in sport – causing tennis elbow (outer side) or golfer's elbow (inner side). You don't have to play golf or tennis to suffer from these problems.

Treatment The problem burns itself out, but can take months. Heat treatment (such as a hot water bottle or heat lamp), gentle massage, a support bandage, and anti-inflammatory drugs like ibuprofen may help. If it's showing no sign of improvement and it's a real nuisance, a cortisone injection may cure it – your GP may do this for you, or refer you on to a specialist. If you do play a club or racquet sport, get some advice about your technique or grip size – minor alterations may solve the problem.

Tenosynovitis Tendons are tough cords which connect muscles to bone. They have a clingfilm-type sheath to help them run smoothly over each other. Repeated movements or exercise which is unusual for you can make these sheaths swell, rub, and become painful. This is tenosynovitis, and it happens most commonly at the wrist.

Treatment When it's caused by exercise you're unaccustomed to, it usually goes away on its own after a few days. Tenosynovitis caused by repetitive movements is more of a problem. Wrist supports, heat, and anti-inflammatories, as for tennis and golfer's elbow, may help; cortisone injections into the tendon sheath can also be very effective, although you'll probably have to see a specialist for this type of treatment. It's important to sort out whatever's causing it. For example, repetitive work with tools, or long hours at the keyboard without breaks or in an awkward position, may

stop the inflamed tendon sheaths from healing. Try to make some simple alterations to your work habits to solve the problem, or discuss the situation with your employer.

Painful arc/frozen shoulder A large cuff of muscles is used in moving your shoulder. If this becomes inflamed – usually for no obvious reason – the shoulder becomes sore and its movements may be restricted. This is known as 'painful arc'. In really severe cases, the pain gets so bad that movement of the shoulder is virtually reduced to zero and the joint is described as being 'frozen'.

Treatment Most of the treatments already discussed for other arm problems will help painful arc, such as heat and anti-inflammatories from the chemist. It's very important to keep the shoulder moving so it doesn't stiffen up too much. One easy way is to do an exercise in which you bend forward slightly and gently swing the arm, at the shoulder, like a pendulum, increasing the movements a little each day. Painful arc and frozen shoulder can take many months – or even a year or two – to settle. Again, a cortisone injection often helps – your GP will be able to arrange this for you. Sometimes, physiotherapy, or even surgery in really severe cases, is the answer, so discuss the situation with your GP if you're getting nowhere.

Trapped nerve The nerves leave the spinal cord, pass through the bones of the neck, and travel through various nooks and crannies before reaching their destinations in the arms. At any point in this journey, they can become trapped. Common areas include the neck, the elbow, and the wrist, and the result is pain and pins and needles or numbness.

Treatment Most trapped nerves free themselves within a day or two. If the problem lasts longer, try anti-inflammatories and gentle exercise. And if this doesn't sort it out, or the problem is severe or quickly getting worse, speak to your GP. The treatment will vary according to where exactly the nerve is trapped, but may involve painkillers, splints, cortisone injections, manipulations and, in occasional persistent and troublesome cases, surgery.

Angina This is explained in the 'Chest pain' section (p. 44). Occasionally, the pain is felt in the left arm as well as – or instead of – in the chest. But remember that it's very unlikely to be the cause of arm pain in the under 45s.

Treatment See the 'Chest pain' section (p. 44).

Back pain

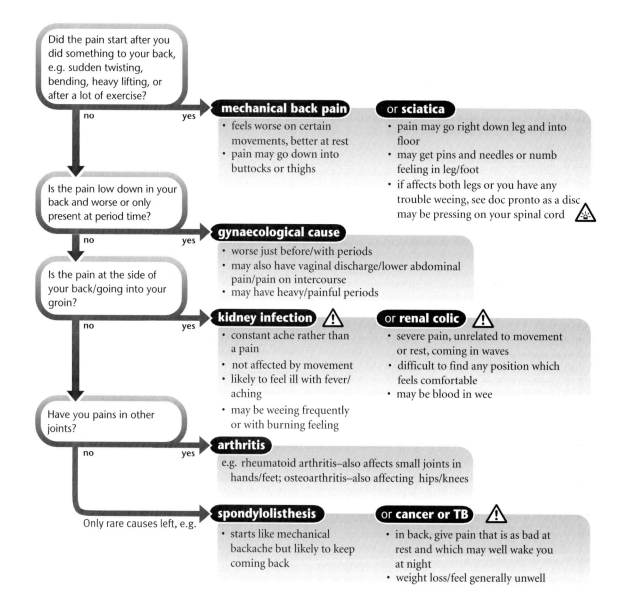

Did the pain start after you did something to your back, e.g. sudden twisting, bending, heavy lifting, or after a lot of exercise?

no → yes →

mechanical back pain
- feels worse on certain movements, better at rest
- pain may go down into buttocks or thighs

or **sciatica**
- pain may go right down leg and into floor
- may get pins and needles or numb feeling in leg/foot
- if affects both legs or you have any trouble weeing, see doc pronto as a disc may be pressing on your spinal cord

Is the pain low down in your back and worse or only present at period time?

no → yes →

gynaecological cause
- worse just before/with periods
- may also have vaginal discharge/lower abdominal pain/pain on intercourse
- may have heavy/painful periods

Is the pain at the side of your back/going into your groin?

no → yes →

kidney infection
- constant ache rather than a pain
- not affected by movement
- likely to feel ill with fever/aching
- may be weeing frequently or with burning feeling

or **renal colic**
- severe pain, unrelated to movement or rest, coming in waves
- difficult to find any position which feels comfortable
- may be blood in wee

Have you pains in other joints?

no → yes →

arthritis
e.g. rheumatoid arthritis–also affects small joints in hands/feet; osteoarthritis–also affecting hips/knees

Only rare causes left, e.g.

spondylolisthesis
- starts like mechanical backache but likely to keep coming back

or **cancer or TB**
- in back, give pain that is as bad at rest and which may well wake you at night
- weight loss/feel generally unwell

Mechanical back pain The back is made up of inter-locking bits (muscles, bones, joints, discs, ligaments, and tendons), that it's pretty much impossible to be totally specific about which bit you've strained or inflamed. And it really doesn't matter anyway because they're all treated in much the same way – so they're lumped together under the blanket term 'mechanical back pain'.

Treatment The days of strict bedrest are long gone. There are two main areas to focus on. First, relieve the pain. The chemist can help with painkillers: anti-inflammatory drugs (e.g. ibuprofen) or paracetamol/codeine mixtures are usu-ally effective. Heat and massage may also help ease the pain, especially if you have a lot of spasm – a cramp-type con-traction of the muscles of your back. Second, get your back moving. Getting up and about, so long as you avoid heavy lifting, twisting, and so on, will help your back heal, even if it feels a bit more painful to begin with. Going swimming is ideal exercise. And stay optimistic: whatever treatment you have, you've an 80–90% chance of the problem being better within six to eight weeks. It's important to get back to work as soon as possible, even if your back doesn't feel 100%. If you're not noticing any signs of improvement after a week or two, consider seeing an osteopath as manipulation may speed things up. And don't expect your doctor to arrange an X-ray of your back, as it's very unlikely to help.

If you get repeated episodes of mechanical pain, then try some preventive measures. These include: dieting if you're overweight; doing gentle back exercises and swimming reg-ularly; being careful with your posture and with lifting; and using a firm mattress.

Sciatica Between each bone which makes up the verte-bral column is a shock absorber known as an intervertebral disc. If one of these shifts sideways, or leaks some fluid, it can irritate a nearby nerve – commonly the sciatic nerve, which runs down the back of your leg. Hence, 'sciatica' or 'slipped disc'.

Treatment Much the same as for mechanical pain. As the pain can be severe, you may need something prescribed by your GP if over-the-counter medicines aren't strong enough. Very occasionally, the problem doesn't settle down or the nerve is quite badly damaged, in which case your GP is likely to refer you to an orthopaedic surgeon to see if surgery might help. Very rarely a slipped disc can press on the spinal cord giving pain down both legs and trouble peeing. This is an urgent hospital job.

Gynaecological cause Pain felt in the back can arise from the pelvic organs – the womb and the ovaries. The obvious example is period pain. Some gynaecological dis-eases such as pelvic inflammatory disease and endometriosis can cause back pain which is worse – or only present – at the time of your periods. Mechanical back pain (see above) may also be aggravated by your periods, either because the hor-monal cycle 'loosens' the ligaments holding the small bones of your spine together, or because your tolerance to the pain is lowered, or both. And a very severe womb prolapse can result in back pain, especially on standing.

Treatment Back pain as a part of period pain is quite normal – its treatment is discussed in the 'Primary dysmenor-rhoea' part of the 'Painful periods' section (p. 114). The treatment of prolapse is covered in the 'Waterworks problems' section (p. 160) and that of pelvic inflammatory disease and endometriosis in the 'Lower abdominal pain – recurrent' section (p. 94).

Kidney infection A germ in the kidney.

Treatment Drink plenty of fluids and see your GP – you will need a course of antibiotics. You may also need some tests to see why you've developed this infection. Your own doctor may arrange these or she may refer you to hospital.

Renal colic This is a stone (usually like a small piece of gravel) in the tube joining the kidney to the bladder. This tube is very thin and muscular, and squeezes hard to push the stone through, causing horrendous pain.

Treatment It probably depends who it's quickest to get to – the local hospital or your GP. You'll be in so much pain you won't really care who sees you, you'll just want it sorted out asap. It needs strong painkillers, usually by injection, and a high fluid intake. If your GP does treat you, she may need to send you to hospital anyway if it doesn't quickly set-tle down. And one way or another, if it's your first attack, you're likely to need further tests.

Arthritis Various types of arthritis, such as rheumatoid arthritis or osteoarthritis, can cause back pain. These are explained further, and their treatment discussed, in the 'Multiple joint pains' (p. 100) and 'Knee pain' (p. 86) sections.

Spondylolisthesis This is a shift forward of one of the bones of the vertebral column on the one underneath.

Treatment Most just require painkillers and the usual back advice outlined above. If the shift is large, or the pain pro-longed and severe, then surgery may be the only answer.

Rare serious causes There's a whole heap of small-print stuff, including cancers, collapse of spinal bones through bone thinning (osteoporosis), some types of arthritis, and bone infection, which can cause back pain. Fortunately, they're all incredibly rare.

Treatment If you think you have a rare serious cause, according to the flow chart, see your GP. If she thinks so too – unlikely – she'll arrange tests or a specialist's opinion.

Bad breath

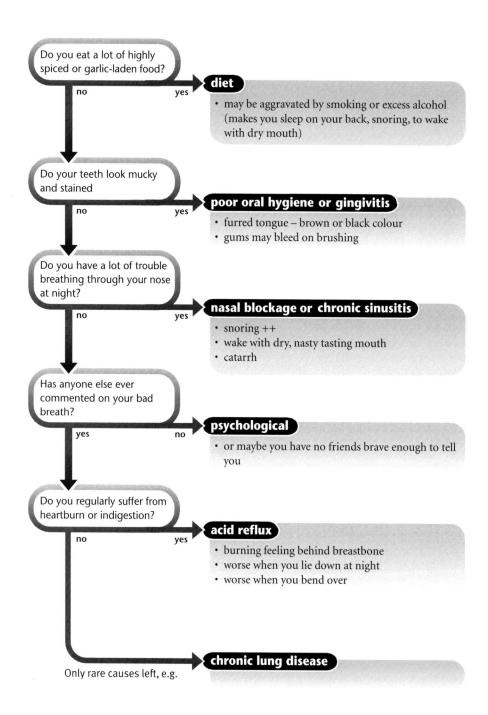

Do you eat a lot of highly spiced or garlic-laden food?

no   yes

diet
- may be aggravated by smoking or excess alcohol (makes you sleep on your back, snoring, to wake with dry mouth)

Do your teeth look mucky and stained

no   yes

poor oral hygiene or gingivitis
- furred tongue – brown or black colour
- gums may bleed on brushing

Do you have a lot of trouble breathing through your nose at night?

no   yes

nasal blockage or chronic sinusitis
- snoring ++
- wake with dry, nasty tasting mouth
- catarrh

Has anyone else ever commented on your bad breath?

yes   no

psychological
- or maybe you have no friends brave enough to tell you

Do you regularly suffer from heartburn or indigestion?

no   yes

acid reflux
- burning feeling behind breastbone
- worse when you lie down at night
- worse when you bend over

chronic lung disease

Only rare causes left, e.g.

Poor oral hygiene Mouth neglect is far and away the most common cause of persistent bad breath ('halitosis'). Unsavoury muck collecting around your teeth and gums – or on your tongue – festers, releasing a smell.

Treatment Regular brushing and flossing will keep your breath fresh smelling. But don't forget your tongue, because a dirty tongue is basically a swamp of microscopic bits of decaying food. A little known trick involves scrubbing the tongue regularly with a soft toothbrush. Push it forward as you do this, or you'll retch and rather spoil the effect. Mouthwashes and breath fresheners may help, but remember they're only cosmetic and don't get to the root of the problem. Saliva is a natural mouthwash which you can stimulate by chewing gum (sugar-free, of course). Also, drink plenty of fluids and swill your mouth with water regularly to dislodge any stuck food particles.

Diet You don't need a medical degree to realize that last night's garlic-drenched creation may put people off entering your personal space for a day or two.

Treatment You could avoid highly spiced foods, but it's more realistic just to put up with the problem until your breath is sweet smelling again after a day or so – or use breath fresheners or mouthwashes to camouflage the problem.

Gingivitis This means infected gums and is usually caused by poor oral hygiene, as outlined above.

Treatment This needs a mouthwash or antibiotics, which your dentist can provide. He ought to give your teeth the once-over anyway, as you've probably been neglecting them, and can give you advice on how to keep your teeth and gums healthy in the future.

Nasal blockage or chronic sinusitis Anything which permanently blocks your nose – such as hay fever, a constantly runny nose, or polyps – will make you snore and breathe through your mouth (see the 'Blocked nose' section, p. 32). As a result, your mouth tends to dry out and this, in turn, causes bad breath. Chronic sinusitis is explained in the 'Hoarse voice' section (p. 76). The dripping of catarrh down the back of the throat can cause bad breath, especially if the catarrh contains certain types of germs.

Treatment If you have to breathe through your mouth all the time because your nose is stuffed up, then you have to sort out whatever's causing the blockage if you want to cure your bad breath. This means a trip to your GP. You'll probably end up with either nose sprays or an appointment for an Ear, Nose, and Throat ('ENT') surgeon for possible surgery. A course of antibiotics may help chronic sinusitis – but usually only for a while. Again, it's a question of sorting out your blocked nose (as in the 'Chronic sinusitis' part of the 'Hoarse voice' section, p. 76), otherwise it's likely to keep coming back.

Psychological You might find that the problem is more in your mind than in your mouth. Some people are simply self-conscious, and become very aware of minor problems with their breath which others would accept as normal. This is just an aspect of their personality and doesn't usually cause a great problem. But if you are depressed or suffering from severe anxiety, you might focus on your breath, becoming convinced that it stinks, despite the fact that no one else ever notices a problem.

Treatment If you think it's possible you're just worrying unnecessarily, your best bet is simply to ask someone who you can trust to give you a straight answer. At least you'll then know whether you've been worrying over nothing, or whether you've got a problem, which you can then get sorted out as described above. If you're suffering badly with anxiety, or you – or friends or family – think you might be depressed, then follow the advice given in the 'Feeling tense' (p. 64) and 'Feeling down' (p. 62) sections.

Acid reflux This is explained, and the treatment outlined, in the 'Indigestion' section (p. 78). Acid, and the stomach contents, coming up into the gullet can release a smell causing bad breath.

Lung disease Any lung disease which produces a lot of infected catarrh can cause bad breath, simply because you'll keep coughing up nasty-smelling phlegm. This is very rarely the cause of halitosis though – especially if your chest isn't really giving you major problems.

Treatment See your GP to get the lung trouble sorted out.

Bleeding from the back passage

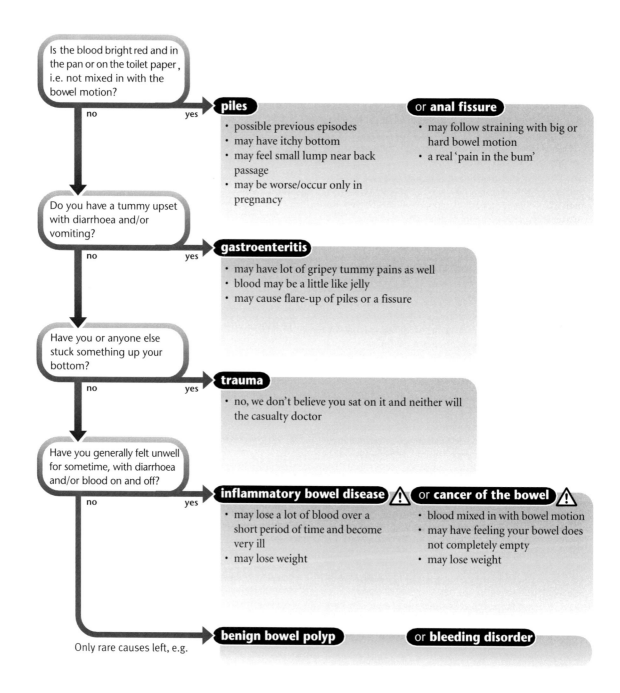

Is the blood bright red and in the pan or on the toilet paper, i.e. not mixed in with the bowel motion?

no — yes →

piles
- possible previous episodes
- may have itchy bottom
- may feel small lump near back passage
- may be worse/occur only in pregnancy

or anal fissure
- may follow straining with big or hard bowel motion
- a real 'pain in the bum'

Do you have a tummy upset with diarrhoea and/or vomiting?

no — yes →

gastroenteritis
- may have lot of gripey tummy pains as well
- blood may be a little like jelly
- may cause flare-up of piles or a fissure

Have you or anyone else stuck something up your bottom?

no — yes →

trauma
- no, we don't believe you sat on it and neither will the casualty doctor

Have you generally felt unwell for sometime, with diarrhoea and/or blood on and off?

no — yes →

inflammatory bowel disease ⚠
- may lose a lot of blood over a short period of time and become very ill
- may lose weight

or cancer of the bowel ⚠
- blood mixed in with bowel motion
- may have feeling your bowel does not completely empty
- may lose weight

Only rare causes left, e.g. →

benign bowel polyp

or bleeding disorder

Remember: ⚠ means see your GP sharpish; ⚠ means an urgent hospital job

Piles These are varicose veins (swollen veins full of blood) in your back passage. They are usually caused by constipation – straining when you go to the toilet tends to make the veins swell. Pregnancy can also be a cause, or will tend to make existing piles worse. They often leak some blood, which you'll notice in the toilet or on the paper when you wipe yourself. They aren't usually painful unless they strangulate – this means that they're being throttled by the muscle of your anus, causing severe pain, increased swelling, and more bleeding.

Treatment Piles will often sort themselves out, especially if you can avoid straining when you go to the toilet. Constipation is usually helped by increasing your fibre and fluid intake, and doing more physical exercise. You can kick-start the process by using a laxative from the chemist, but these are probably best kept to a minimum. It's also important not to spend too long in the loo, as the posture of sitting on the toilet actually makes the problem worse – so no reading while you're in there. And don't ignore the early morning urge to go to the toilet, no matter how pushed you are for time. Creams from the chemist will help any irritation the piles are causing, but will make no difference to the bleeding. If you keep getting problems, see your GP – she may refer you to a surgeon for a small operation which should solve the problem. You'll need urgent treatment if your piles have strangulated. The pain will normally get you to your GP pretty quickly.

Anal fissure This is a split in the back passage. Again, constipation is the likely cause; straining to pass a large motion causes the split, which then leaks some blood. It can also start after an attack of diarrhoea.

Treatment Most fissures heal themselves quickly. The advice already given about constipation (see above) is vital. Fissures are painful, so it's tempting to avoid going to the toilet. If you do this, you'll get more constipated, with the risk of opening up the split again when you do go – so get those bowels opening regularly and easily. Keep the tail end clean to give the fissure a chance to heal: carry around a small pack of wet-wipes so you can clean up thoroughly and painlessly each time you go to the toilet. Creams from the chemist usually help ease the pain. If you seem to be getting nowhere, see your GP – she can prescribe alternative creams or refer you to a surgeon for a small operation if all else fails.

Gastroenteritis This is explained in the 'Abdominal pain – one-off' (p. 8) and 'Diarrhoea' (p. 50) sections. One particular germ – 'campylobacter' – can inflame the bowel so much that it causes bleeding.

Treatment See the 'Abdominal pain' section. If the bleeding happens a few times, it's worth contacting your GP. He may want to check you out for the Campylobacter germ because antibiotics may get you better quicker.

Inflammatory bowel disease This is explained, and the treatment outlined, in the 'Diarrhoea' section (p. 50).

Trauma Nature did not intend anything to be poked up the backside. It's not surprising, then, that sticking objects in your rear end can cause some damage, resulting in bleeding. Anal sex is the likeliest culprit.

Treatment Unless the bleeding is very insignificant and painless, it's best to get to casualty to check how much damage has been done.

Cancer This is very unlikely in the under 40s. For further details, see the 'Diarrhoea' section (p. 50).

Rare causes A few rarities like polyps in the bowel (which sometimes run in families) and bleeding disorders (problems with your blood clotting) can cause bleeding from the back passage.

Treatment See your GP – if she thinks you might have a rare problem like this, she'll get it checked out.

Blisters

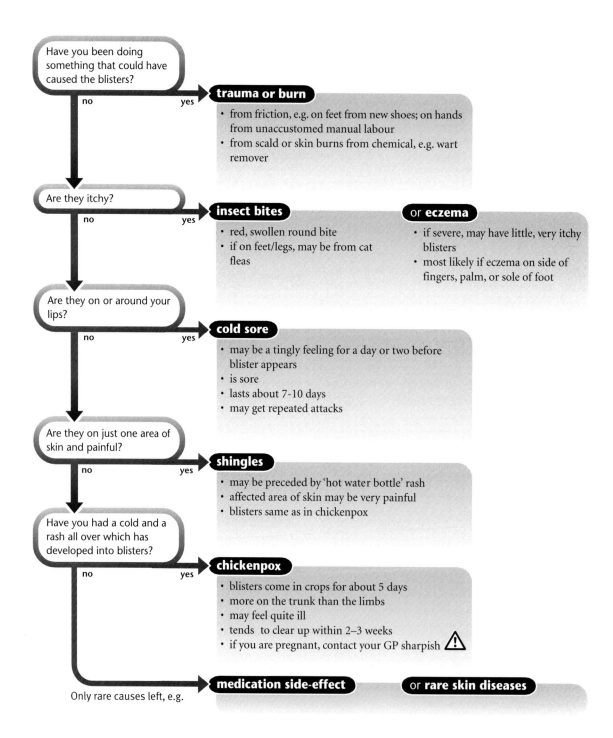

Have you been doing something that could have caused the blisters?

no / yes

trauma or burn
- from friction, e.g. on feet from new shoes; on hands from unaccustomed manual labour
- from scald or skin burns from chemical, e.g. wart remover

Are they itchy?

no / yes

insect bites
- red, swollen round bite
- if on feet/legs, may be from cat fleas

or eczema
- if severe, may have little, very itchy blisters
- most likely if eczema on side of fingers, palm, or sole of foot

Are they on or around your lips?

no / yes

cold sore
- may be a tingly feeling for a day or two before blister appears
- is sore
- lasts about 7-10 days
- may get repeated attacks

Are they on just one area of skin and painful?

no / yes

shingles
- may be preceded by 'hot water bottle' rash
- affected area of skin may be very painful
- blisters same as in chickenpox

Have you had a cold and a rash all over which has developed into blisters?

no / yes

chickenpox
- blisters come in crops for about 5 days
- more on the trunk than the limbs
- may feel quite ill
- tends to clear up within 2–3 weeks
- if you are pregnant, contact your GP sharpish ⚠

Only rare causes left, e.g.

medication side-effect   **or rare skin diseases**

Trauma Everyone is familiar with blisters on the feet caused by new shoes or a long walk or run. The cause is friction, which leads to a build-up of fluid under the skin. Similar blisters can also develop after a burn.

Treatment Friction blisters settle down quickly and don't need any treatment except maybe a change of shoe and a protective plaster. A burn may take longer to heal – if you're worried, get it checked by the nurse at your practice to make sure it doesn't need any special dressings or antibiotics. Usually, it's better to leave blisters alone rather than deliberately burst them.

Insect bites These are discussed, and their treatment outlined, in the 'Itchy skin' section (p. 84). They can sometimes result in quite large blisters. If you keep getting problems with insect bites, try to work out – and sort out – wherever they're coming from. Likely sources include pets (dogs, cats, and birds) and bedding or furniture.

Cold sore See the 'Rash on the face' section (p. 128).

Eczema One type of eczema – 'pompholyx' – can cause tiny, itchy blisters on the palms and sides of the fingers. The same pattern can also develop on the feet. Other forms of eczema can also develop blisters when they're flaring up or infected. For more information on eczema, see the 'Itchy skin' section (p. 84).

Treatment Mild pompholyx may be helped by a moisturizer and hydrocortisone 1% cream from the chemist. It's important to avoid things which might irritate your skin such as detergents and strong soaps. Often, though, this problem will need stronger treatments, in which case your GP can help. You'll also need to see her if you have any other type of eczema which has flared up so badly that it's caused blisters.

Shingles Once you've had chickenpox, the virus which causes it never fully leaves your system – it lies dormant somewhere in your spine. In the future, for no obvious reason, it can reactivate, resulting in shingles.

Treatment Shingles goes away on its own over a few weeks. The blisters become weepy, then scab over, and finally heal. Usually, the only treatment needed is nothing more than painkillers and dressings from the chemist. It's worth steering clear of women who are (or are trying to get) pregnant while you have the rash. This is because when you have shingles it's possible to pass the virus on to anyone who's never had chickenpox before, and this can damage a developing baby – although the risk is very small.

There are lots of old wives' tales about shingles, but they're all nonsense. The only times it can really be troublesome are if you already have some problem which weakens your immune system (such as being on high-dose steroid tablets or chemotherapy drugs for cancer) or if shingles affects the area around your eye (it can get into the eye itself, causing complications). In both cases, contact your GP urgently.

Some doctors prescribe a certain type of medication in shingles, but this is only really useful in the elderly or in the special situations outlined above – and then only if started very soon after the rash first appears. Occasionally, the pain of shingles can carry on long after the rash has gone – this is known as post-herpetic neuralgia. Again, this only usually affects the elderly. It can be treated quite effectively, so if you think you have this problem, discuss the situation with your GP.

Chickenpox (and other viruses) Viruses can cause all sorts of rashes (as well as other typical symptoms like a fever and sore throat) – sometimes these result in blisters, the most well-known example being chickenpox.

Treatment Usually, these viruses don't require any special treatment other than the paracetamol and fluids you'd normally take for a cold or flu. If you get chickenpox, you may feel pretty unwell – rest, and use calamine lotion to ease the itch. You'll need to contact your GP if you already have a weakened immune system (see 'Shingles' above) or if you're becoming increasingly unwell, especially if you develop a bad cough or breathlessness (the virus can occasionally affect the lungs). The advice given under 'Shingles' about avoiding pregnant women applies too. If you are (or think you might be) pregnant and you're developing chickenpox then you need to get in touch with your GP urgently, as it may cause you or your baby some problems.

Medication side-effect Some prescribed treatments can cause blisters as a side-effect, though it's pretty unlikely that you'll be taking any of them.

Treatment If you think your blisters might be caused by your medication, discuss the situation with whoever prescribed them.

Rare skin disorders Some very small-print skin diseases can cause unexplained blisters which may keep coming back.

Treatment See your GP – if she thinks you've got an unusual skin disease, she'll arrange for you to see a dermatologist (skin specialist).

Blocked nose

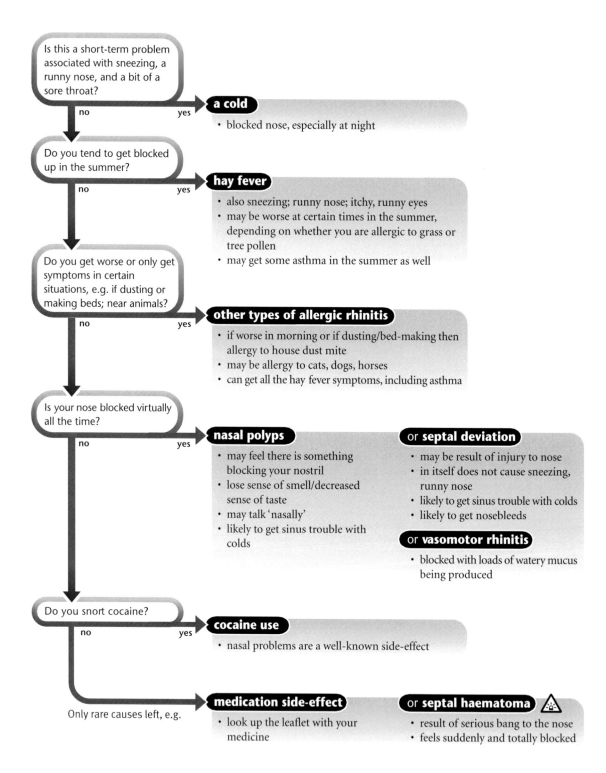

Is this a short-term problem associated with sneezing, a runny nose, and a bit of a sore throat?

yes → **a cold**
- blocked nose, especially at night

no ↓

Do you tend to get blocked up in the summer?

yes → **hay fever**
- also sneezing; runny nose; itchy, runny eyes
- may be worse at certain times in the summer, depending on whether you are allergic to grass or tree pollen
- may get some asthma in the summer as well

no ↓

Do you get worse or only get symptoms in certain situations, e.g. if dusting or making beds; near animals?

yes → **other types of allergic rhinitis**
- if worse in morning or if dusting/bed-making then allergy to house dust mite
- may be allergy to cats, dogs, horses
- can get all the hay fever symptoms, including asthma

no ↓

Is your nose blocked virtually all the time?

yes → **nasal polyps**
- may feel there is something blocking your nostril
- lose sense of smell/decreased sense of taste
- may talk 'nasally'
- likely to get sinus trouble with colds

or septal deviation
- may be result of injury to nose
- in itself does not cause sneezing, runny nose
- likely to get sinus trouble with colds
- likely to get nosebleeds

or vasomotor rhinitis
- blocked with loads of watery mucus being produced

no ↓

Do you snort cocaine?

yes → **cocaine use**
- nasal problems are a well-known side-effect

Only rare causes left, e.g. → **medication side-effect**
- look up the leaflet with your medicine

or septal haematoma
- result of serious bang to the nose
- feels suddenly and totally blocked

A cold Your nose reacts to the virus which causes colds by making more catarrh to prevent any more germs getting into your system. The result: the familiar bunged-up nose.

Treatment There's no point seeing your GP about a cold because there's no magic cure. Just take plenty of fluids and paracetamol for the headache or sore throat which goes with the cold. The stuffed-up feeling may be helped by steam inhalations.

Hay fever This is an allergy to pollen which inflames the inside of your nose and throat. The glands in your nose go into overdrive, producing loads of mucus, which results in a runny, blocked nose and sneezing.

Treatment Simple measures include avoiding long walks when the pollen count is high (usually early morning and evening), and keeping the car windows wound up (otherwise the car acts as a pollen trap). Further advice about eye problems caused by hay fever are given in the 'Red eye' section (p. 130). Have a word with your chemist – a lot of effective hay fever treatment is now available over the counter, including antihistamine tablets and steroid nose sprays. If you're getting nowhere, see your GP. She may try other antihistamines or nose sprays or, if you're really bad, she may even use steroids in the form of a course of tablets or a 'one-off' injection.

Other types of allergic rhinitis You may be allergic to something other than pollen, resulting in stuffy-nosed misery very similar to hay fever ('rhinitis'). Your symptoms may only happen in specific situations (e.g. cat allergy) or may be there much of the time (e.g. house dust mite allergy).

Treatment If you can, avoid whatever you're allergic to. Allergy tests aren't usually much help – it's either obvious what the allergy is or, if not, then it's usually something you can't really avoid anyway (such as house dust – although, in this case, bear in mind that feather pillows act as a dust trap, so using foam ones may help). Effective treatments such as antihistamines and steroid nose sprays are available from the chemist.

Vasomotor rhinitis This makes your nose produce loads of watery catarrh which can leak out like water from a tap. It's possibly caused by leaky blood vessels in the nose.

Treatment Steroid nose sprays are worth a try, although they may not work as well as in the allergic types of rhinitis. Otherwise, see your GP, who may prescribe other types of nose spray. Surgery can be considered if you're really desperate.

Nasal polyps These are fleshy bits of gristle which can grow inside your nose, blocking the airway. They are more common in people with allergic rhinitis or asthma.

Treatment Steroid nose sprays from the chemist can shrink polyps down enough to ease the block. If you're getting nowhere and you'd consider surgery, see your GP, who may refer you to an Ear, Nose, and Throat ('ENT') specialist – polyps can be cut out, although they can come back again in the future.

Cocaine use Sniffing up naughty substances can cause some damage, leading to a drippy and blocked nose.

Treatment Easy – avoid snorting cocaine.

Septal deviation The nasal septum is the bony bit in the middle of your nose separating your two nostrils. It can bend to one side or the other, causing a blockage. This is usually the result of an old injury – or maybe you were born with it.

Treatment The only way to cure this is with surgery. So if the problem is bad enough, speak to your GP, who will refer you to an ENT surgeon.

Medication side-effect Some treatments – either prescribed or over-the-counter – can cause a blocked nose. For example, certain types of spray used for blocked noses and sinusitis (available from the chemist) cause a 'rebound' effect: this means they help while you use them, but when you stop, the stuffiness can return worse than it was in the first place. As a result, some people end up using the spray constantly because the problem gets much worse whenever they stop. Some blood pressure pills prescribed by your GP also have the side-effect of causing a blocked-up nose.

Treatment If you think an over-the-counter spray may be making you worse, speak to your chemist or GP. And if you're on prescribed treatment, check the leaflet in the pack – if a blocked or runny nose is mentioned as a side-effect, see your GP as she may be able to stop the treatment or prescribe you something else instead.

Septal haematoma This is a large bruise of the nasal septum (see above). The internal swelling it causes is so large that it blocks the nose. It's rare, but occasionally results from a serious thump on the nose.

Treatment Go to casualty. The blood which causes the internal swelling needs to be drained off, otherwise your nose can end up with permanent damage.

Blood in spit

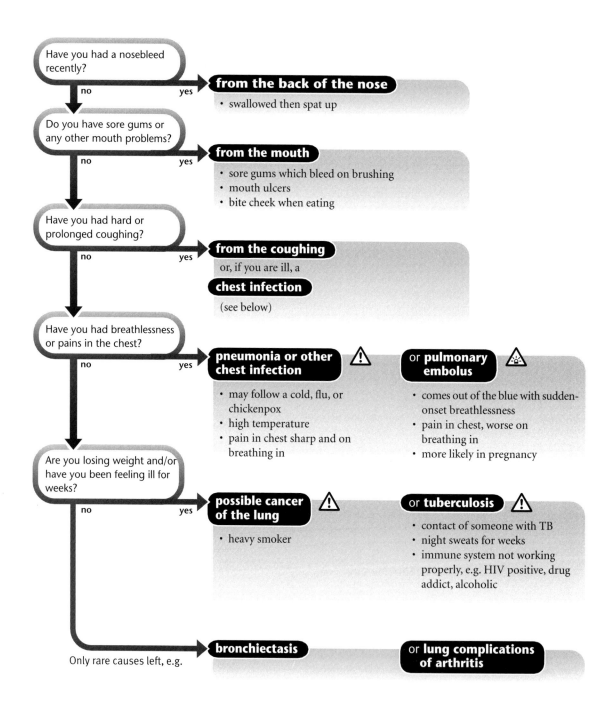

Have you had a nosebleed recently?

no — yes →

from the back of the nose
- swallowed then spat up

Do you have sore gums or any other mouth problems?

no — yes →

from the mouth
- sore gums which bleed on brushing
- mouth ulcers
- bite cheek when eating

Have you had hard or prolonged coughing?

no — yes →

from the coughing
or, if you are ill, a
chest infection
(see below)

Have you had breathlessness or pains in the chest?

no — yes →

pneumonia or other chest infection ⚠
- may follow a cold, flu, or chickenpox
- high temperature
- pain in chest sharp and on breathing in

or pulmonary embolus ⚠
- comes out of the blue with sudden-onset breathlessness
- pain in chest, worse on breathing in
- more likely in pregnancy

Are you losing weight and/or have you been feeling ill for weeks?

no — yes →

possible cancer of the lung ⚠
- heavy smoker

or tuberculosis ⚠
- contact of someone with TB
- night sweats for weeks
- immune system not working properly, e.g. HIV positive, drug addict, alcoholic

Only rare causes left, e.g.

bronchiectasis

or lung complications of arthritis

Remember: ⚠ means see your GP sharpish; ⚠ means an urgent hospital job

Hard or prolonged coughing If you cough long or hard enough, whatever the cause of the cough, you can rupture a small blood vessel in your windpipe. Blood will leak into your spit, which you then cough up. As the blood vessel heals up, the bleeding stops.

Treatment There's no specific treatment needed – usually the blood only appears in your phlegm once or twice before it all settles down. Otherwise, all you need to do is treat whatever's causing the cough, which is probably a virus infection of your throat and windpipe. There's no magic cure – just try steam inhalations, plenty of fluids, and avoid cigarette smoke. If you're coughing green or yellow phlegm and you feel ill, breathless, or feverish, you may need antibiotics, so discuss the situation with your GP.

From a nosebleed or from the mouth Blood from a nosebleed can drip back into the throat and then be coughed up. The same can happen to blood from the mouth (such as a cut or bleeding gums).

Treatment These situations are harmless and don't need any particular treatment.

Pneumonia A severe form of chest infection. See 'Cough' section (p. 46).

Treatment This is covered in the 'Cough' section (p. 46).

Pulmonary embolus This is a blood clot in the lung. It usually forms somewhere else in the body and is carried in the circulation to the lungs, where it blocks a blood vessel. As a result, a small part of the lung is starved of oxygen, causing pain, breathlessness, and blood in the spit. Very occasionally, it can be caused by blood clots forming in the leg veins, which can happen if you've not used your leg muscles for a while (e.g. during a long-haul flight or when your leg's in plaster) or during (or shortly after) pregnancy; it's a bit more common (though still rare) in women on the Pill.

Treatment A definite hospital job. A bad one will leave you in no doubt what to do because the symptoms will be severe – call an ambulance. They can be more subtle though. If in real doubt, get advice from your GP. If you've had a pulmonary embolus then you shouln't use the Pill for family planning any more, as this raises the chances of another one.

Tuberculosis TB is an infection of the lung caused by a particular germ which can make you very unwell and can be difficult to treat. It is rare these days, though does sometimes occur, especially in immigrants.

Treatment Your first stop is likely to be your GP. After tests, especially an X-ray of your chest, she will refer you to the local chest consultant for specialized treatment.

Lung cancer This is very rare under the age of 40. The blood vessels supplying the cancer can leak, causing repeated episodes of blood in the spit, which is how this type of cancer may first show itself.

Treatment As for tuberculosis – a chest X-ray will show a shadow and the specialist will arrange further tests to confirm the diagnosis, and will then plan your treatment. This is likely to involve surgery (to remove the cancer), radiotherapy (treatment with radiation rays), or chemotherapy (treatment with powerful drugs).

Other medical rarities There are a number of unusual medical conditions which can reveal themselves by causing bloodstained spit. Some affect only the lung (such as bronchiectasis – a constantly infected and damaged part of the lung) and others affect other parts of the body (such as some unusual joint diseases).

Treatment You are highly unlikely to be affected by any of these conditions – see your GP if you want the problem checked out.

Blood in urine

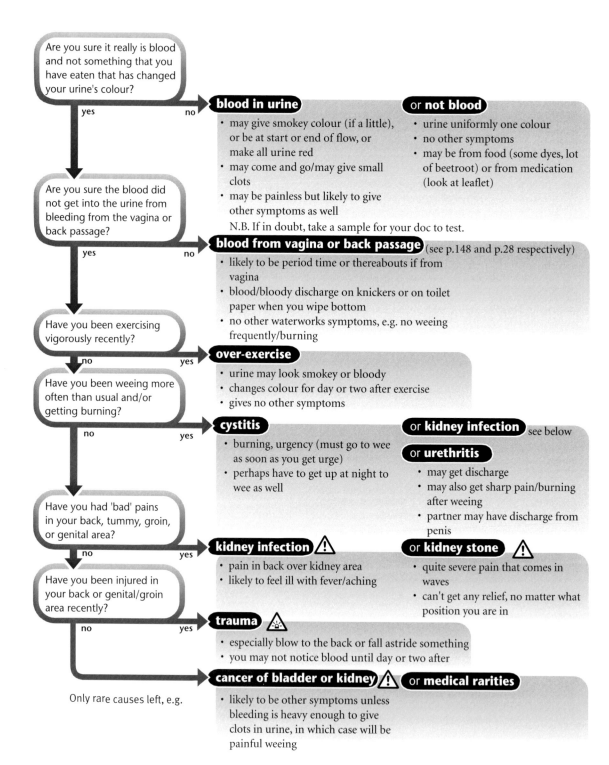

Are you sure it really is blood and not something that you have eaten that has changed your urine's colour?

yes / no

blood in urine
- may give smokey colour (if a little), or be at start or end of flow, or make all urine red
- may come and go/may give small clots
- may be painless but likely to give other symptoms as well

N.B. If in doubt, take a sample for your doc to test.

or not blood
- urine uniformly one colour
- no other symptoms
- may be from food (some dyes, lot of beetroot) or from medication (look at leaflet)

Are you sure the blood did not get into the urine from bleeding from the vagina or back passage?

yes / no

blood from vagina or back passage (see p.148 and p.28 respectively)
- likely to be period time or thereabouts if from vagina
- blood/bloody discharge on knickers or on toilet paper when you wipe bottom
- no other waterworks symptoms, e.g. no weeing frequently/burning

Have you been exercising vigorously recently?

no / yes

over-exercise
- urine may look smokey or bloody
- changes colour for day or two after exercise
- gives no other symptoms

Have you been weeing more often than usual and/or getting burning?

no / yes

cystitis
- burning, urgency (must go to wee as soon as you get urge)
- perhaps have to get up at night to wee as well

or kidney infection see below

or urethritis
- may get discharge
- may also get sharp pain/burning after weeing
- partner may have discharge from penis

Have you had 'bad' pains in your back, tummy, groin, or genital area?

no / yes

kidney infection ⚠
- pain in back over kidney area
- likely to feel ill with fever/aching

or kidney stone ⚠
- quite severe pain that comes in waves
- can't get any relief, no matter what position you are in

Have you been injured in your back or genital/groin area recently?

no / yes

trauma ⚠
- especially blow to the back or fall astride something
- you may not notice blood until day or two after

Only rare causes left, e.g.

cancer of bladder or kidney ⚠ **or medical rarities**
- likely to be other symptoms unless bleeding is heavy enough to give clots in urine, in which case will be painful weeing

Cystitis This is explained in the 'Waterworks problems' section (p. 160). The infection can inflame your bladder so much that it leaks blood.

Kidney infection This is explained in the 'Back pain' section (p. 24).

Kidney stone Stones, like bits of gravel, can develop in your kidney (which makes your urine) or your bladder (which stores it). The irritation they cause can lead to bleeding, so blood appears in your wee. This can also happen if the stone travels down the tube leading from the kidney to bladder (the 'ureter'), which is usually very painful (see the 'Renal colic' part of the 'Back pain' section, p. 24).

Treatment See the 'Back pain' (p. 24) and 'Waterworks problems' (p. 160) sections for advice on treating kidney and bladder stones.

Over-exercise A really long road-run or similar exercise on a hard surface can leave you 'weeing blood'. Except it isn't really blood at all. The red blood cells simply get mashed up when they pass through the blood vessels in your pounding feet. This makes them leak their pigment, which is passed out in your urine and can look just like blood.

Treatment This is harmless, so long as it doesn't keep happening whenever you exercise (in which case it can cause anaemia). But if you're not absolutely sure this is the cause, or you feel ill, you need to see a doctor – and try to take a specimen of urine for her to test.

Urethritis A sexually transmitted germ can inflame your urethra to the point that it leaks a little blood when you wee.

Treatment See the 'Urethritis' part of the 'Waterworks problems' section (p. 160).

Trauma Some injuries can result in blood appearing in your urine. For example, a fall astride the frame of your bike might damage your urethra. The kidneys can also be bruised or damaged – for example, by a kick or punch to the loin (the area each side of your lower back between the lowest part of your ribs and the highest part of your pelvis).

Treatment If you see blood in your wee after an injury, go straight to casualty as you may have done some serious damage.

(Cancer of the kidney or bladder) Bladder cancers usually show themselves by leaking blood into the urine – but bear in mind that they are very unusual in the under 50s. Kidney cancers are rarer, but can occur in a younger age group (under 40).

Treatment See your GP. If she's worried, she'll refer you to a urologist (waterworks specialist) for further tests.

(Other medical rarities) There are a number of unusual problems which can cause blood in your urine, including glomerulonephritis (inflamed kidneys), polycystic kidneys (swellings on the kidneys, which runs in families), and bleeding disorders (the blood is too thin and doesn't clot properly).

Treatment It's unlikely that you'll have any of these problems. Speak to your GP if you're concerned – she'll arrange any necessary tests.

Breast lumps

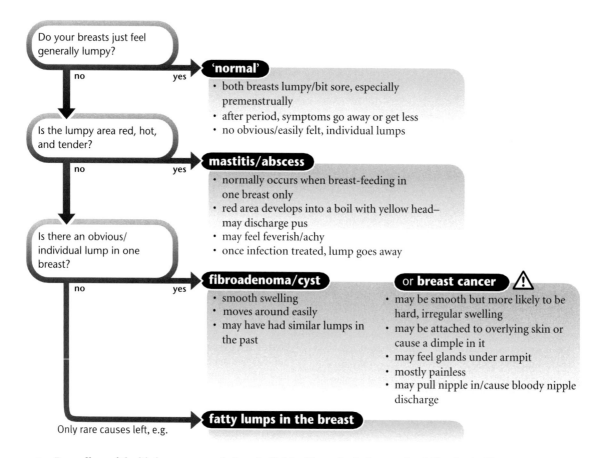

Do your breasts just feel generally lumpy?

no → yes →

'normal'
- both breasts lumpy/bit sore, especially premenstrually
- after period, symptoms go away or get less
- no obvious/easily felt, individual lumps

Is the lumpy area red, hot, and tender?

no → yes →

mastitis/abscess
- normally occurs when breast-feeding in one breast only
- red area develops into a boil with yellow head– may discharge pus
- may feel feverish/achy
- once infection treated, lump goes away

Is there an obvious/ individual lump in one breast?

no → yes →

fibroadenoma/cyst
- smooth swelling
- moves around easily
- may have had similar lumps in the past

or breast cancer ⚠
- may be smooth but more likely to be hard, irregular swelling
- may be attached to overlying skin or cause a dimple in it
- may feel glands under armpit
- mostly painless
- may pull nipple in/cause bloody nipple discharge

Only rare causes left, e.g.

fatty lumps in the breast

⚠ Regardless of the likely cause, any obvious/individual lump in the breast should be checked by your GP as soon as possible.

'Normal' It's quite common for your breasts, at times, to feel 'lumpier' than usual – especially before a period. Also, you might be able to feel your ribs under the breast tissue, which can give the impression of a lump when in fact the breast itself is entirely normal.

Treatment If you can feel a definite lump then this must be checked by your GP. But if it's just a vague lumpiness that you've noticed, try feeling again after your next period. It it's gone then there's nothing to worry about. If not, then there's still probably nothing to worry about, but it's important to get your GP to examine your breasts – she'll refer you to a specialist for a check if there's any doubt that everything's OK. It's worth noting that these days most doctors are less keen on women practising 'ritual' breast self-examination each month. This is because research shows that self-examination, though apparently sensible, is not very good at picking up serious lumps – but it does tend to cause a lot of anxiety by turning up irrelevant and harmless problems. So most doctors now suggest 'breast awareness', which means being generally aware of what your breasts look and feel like so that you'll notice any significant change.

Fibroadenoma This is a harmless gristly lump in the breast which is very common in the 15–30 years age group. It's sometimes called a 'breast mouse' because it is very mobile and slips away from under your fingers when you try to feel it.

Treatment Although this type of lump is not 'malignant' (cancerous) and causes no problems, it still needs to be checked by a breast specialist so that you can be sure it's nothing more serious – so see your GP.

Cyst This is a fluid-filled lump in the breast which is nearly always 'benign' (non-cancerous) and is most common in the 40–50 years age group.

Treatment As for all breast lumps, you need to get this checked by your GP. If she thinks it's a cyst, she may try to sort it out by drawing off the fluid inside the cyst with a needle, or she may refer you to a specialist to get it checked and treated.

Mastitis/abscess These are explained, and the treatments outlined, in the 'Breast pain' section (p. 40).

Breast cancer Cancer of the breast is, thankfully, rare in the under-35 age group.

Treatment See your GP asap – she'll refer you urgently to a breast specialist for assessment and treatment.

Other rare causes There are other unusal causes for lumps in the breast, such as severe bruising and fatty lumps.

Treatment It's unlikely that one of these unusual problems is the cause of your lump – and most are harmless anyway. Nonetheless, you need to get it checked by your GP.

Breast pain

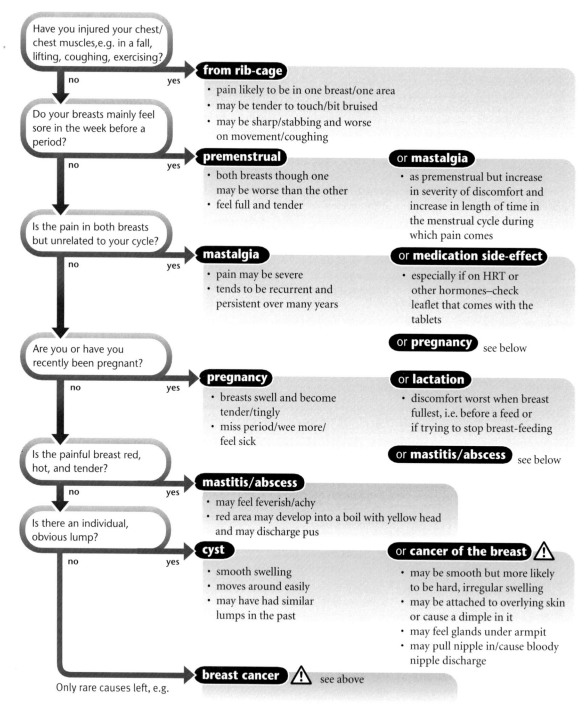

Have you injured your chest/chest muscles, e.g. in a fall, lifting, coughing, exercising?

no → yes

from rib-cage
- pain likely to be in one breast/one area
- may be tender to touch/bit bruised
- may be sharp/stabbing and worse on movement/coughing

Do your breasts mainly feel sore in the week before a period?

no → yes

premenstrual
- both breasts though one may be worse than the other
- feel full and tender

or mastalgia
- as premenstrual but increase in severity of discomfort and increase in length of time in the menstrual cycle during which pain comes

Is the pain in both breasts but unrelated to your cycle?

no → yes

mastalgia
- pain may be severe
- tends to be recurrent and persistent over many years

or medication side-effect
- especially if on HRT or other hormones–check leaflet that comes with the tablets

or pregnancy see below

Are you or have you recently been pregnant?

no → yes

pregnancy
- breasts swell and become tender/tingly
- miss period/wee more/feel sick

or lactation
- discomfort worst when breast fullest, i.e. before a feed or if trying to stop breast-feeding

or mastitis/abscess see below

Is the painful breast red, hot, and tender?

no → yes

mastitis/abscess
- may feel feverish/achy
- red area may develop into a boil with yellow head and may discharge pus

Is there an individual, obvious lump?

no → yes

cyst
- smooth swelling
- moves around easily
- may have had similar lumps in the past

or cancer of the breast ⚠
- may be smooth but more likely to be hard, irregular swelling
- may be attached to overlying skin or cause a dimple in it
- may feel glands under armpit
- may pull nipple in/cause bloody nipple discharge

breast cancer ⚠ see above

Only rare causes left, e.g.

 Regardless of the likely cause, any obvious/individual lump should be checked by your GP as soon as possible.

Breast pain

Premenstrual Your hormonal cycle can make your breasts swell before a period, causing some discomfort. This is common, affecting two out of three women.

Treatment This is quite 'normal' and so is unlikely to need any treatment. If troublesome, a supporting bra, a hot bath, and a mild painkiller should help.

Mastalgia This literally means 'breast pain'. Some women suffer 'cyclical' mastalgia, which is a severe form of 'normal' premenstrual breast pain. Others experience 'non-cyclical' mastalgia, in which the pain is not linked at all with the menstrual cycle. The precise cause is unknown.

Treatment Any breast symptom tends to create the fear of possible serious disease, such as cancer. Fortunately, breast pain is highly unlikely to be caused by anything sinister – if the problem affects both sides or is cyclical you can definitely relax. If it's one-sided, so long as you can't feel a lump you only need get it checked if it's very severe and in one persistent place – and even then it's very unlikely to be anything serious. Mild mastalgia is usually helped by the measures mentioned under 'Premenstrual' above. More severe problems may be helped by anti-inflammatory drugs such as ibuprofen (available over the counter). If you're getting nowhere and the pain is a real problem, see your GP, as she may prescribe you more powerful treatments.

Medication side-effect 'Depot' contraception injections and, occasionally, the Pill and hormone replacement therapy (which you're unlikely to be on unless you're older than 50 or have had an early menopause), can cause breast tenderness.

Treatment Try the measures outlined above. If this doesn't help then discuss the situation with your GP – a change of treatment might do the trick.

From rib-cage A sore rib or a strained muscle can cause a pain which may feel as though it is coming from the breast.

Treatment This will usually go away on its own after a few days. Painkillers and heat (in the form of a hot bath or a heat lamp) may help.

Cyst A cyst is a harmless, fluid-filled lump in the breast, which may be quite sore. For further details, and advice on treatment, see the 'Breast lump' section (p. 38).

Pregnancy The hormone changes caused by early pregnancy make the breasts swell and become tender. Nausea, frequent trips to the loo, and the lack of an expected period may also give the game away.

Treatment This is quite normal and needs no specific treatment. If you're desperate, and hot baths and a supporting bra don't sort the problem out, then you can try paracetamol, which is perfectly safe in pregnancy.

Lactation This is the production of milk by the breasts after childbirth which, not surprisingly, makes the breasts swell and become sore.

Treatment If you're breast-feeding, the pain may be aggravated by the baby chomping on your nipple. Your midwife may be able to give you helpful advice about your feeding technique. Assuming you want to persevere, continue feeding – or at least expressing milk – to relieve the pressure and ensure the milk supply continues. If you want to stop – or not start – breast-feeding, you'll find the discomfort settles after a few days as the milk supply is switched off. The sort of treatments described under 'Premenstrual' (see above) will help.

Mastitis/abscess Mastitis is an infection of the breast, caused by a germ entering through a crack in the nipple – usually in a breast-feeding mother. The infection can develop into a pus-filled lump, known as an abscess.

Treatment See your GP asap. Antibiotics will stop most infections before they cause too much trouble. If you're unlucky and you do end up with an abscess, you'll be sent to hospital to have it lanced under anaesthetic. If you've just had a baby and you want to persevere with breast-feeding, then you need to keep emptying the breast – either by feeding your baby or by expressing the milk – otherwise the milk supply may 'switch off'.

Breast cancer This is highly unlikely to be the cause of your breast pain (see 'Mastalgia' above). Very occasionally, a cancer can cause a persistent, severe pain, usually in one small area of one breast. Roughly one in 37 women who are referred on to a hospital breast unit with breast pain as their major symptom will have cancer (one in 20 with a painful lump).

Treatment See your GP if you're worried that this might be the cause.

Calf pain

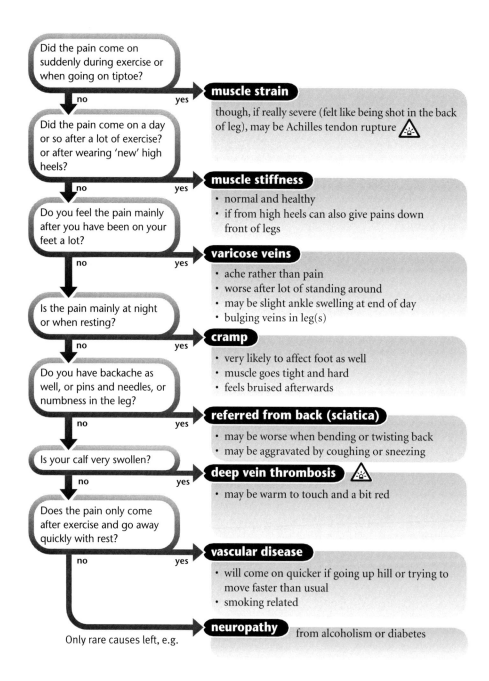

Did the pain come on suddenly during exercise or when going on tiptoe?

no | yes

muscle strain

though, if really severe (felt like being shot in the back of leg), may be Achilles tendon rupture ⚠

Did the pain come on a day or so after a lot of exercise? or after wearing 'new' high heels?

no | yes

muscle stiffness

- normal and healthy
- if from high heels can also give pains down front of legs

Do you feel the pain mainly after you have been on your feet a lot?

no | yes

varicose veins

- ache rather than pain
- worse after lot of standing around
- may be slight ankle swelling at end of day
- bulging veins in leg(s)

Is the pain mainly at night or when resting?

no | yes

cramp

- very likely to affect foot as well
- muscle goes tight and hard
- feels bruised afterwards

Do you have backache as well, or pins and needles, or numbness in the leg?

no | yes

referred from back (sciatica)

- may be worse when bending or twisting back
- may be aggravated by coughing or sneezing

Is your calf very swollen?

no | yes

deep vein thrombosis ⚠

- may be warm to touch and a bit red

Does the pain only come after exercise and go away quickly with rest?

no | yes

vascular disease

- will come on quicker if going up hill or trying to move faster than usual
- smoking related

Only rare causes left, e.g.

neuropathy from alcoholism or diabetes

Remember: ⚠ means see your GP sharpish; ⚠ means an urgent hospital job

Muscle strain If you overstretch a muscle, some of the individual strands which make up the muscle can tear, causing a sudden pain.

Treatment For a bad strain, you may need to rest the calf for a few days and use ice-packs and painkillers (anti-inflammatory tablets such as ibuprofen – available from the chemist – can be particularly useful). Once the strain has healed, you will need to be careful with your normal sporting activities – if you do too much too soon, it'll flare up again. Remember warm-ups and stretching, as described below. A mild strain will get better within a few days and needs no special treatment, a more severe one may take six to eight weeks to heal.

Muscle stiffness (unaccustomed exercise)

Muscles which haven't been used for a while can swell and become sore after a bout of exercise.

Treatment The pain will sort itself out after a day or two. The most you'll need is a simple painkiller like paracetamol. To prevent it happening in the future, improve your level of fitness, building up your exercise gradually, and doing a gentle warm-up and stretching routine before you really get going.

Cramp The calf muscles can go into spasm, causing severe pain at the time and leaving the area with a bruised feeling for a day or two afterwards. It's usually caused by being unfit or overdoing the exercise.

Treatment An attack of cramp can be cured simply by stretching the calf muscle – straighten the affected leg and, with your hand, pull your foot up towards you. Preventive measures include drinking enough fluids (especially before and after exercise), keeping reasonably fit, and warming up before any exertion. Stretching the calf muscles before exercise and bedtime will also prevent cramp – stretch the muscle a few times, just as you would for an attack of cramp. If all else fails and it's becoming a real problem, speak to your GP – sometimes tablets can help.

Referred from back Referred pain is pain which comes from one area but is felt in another. Back trouble – especially 'sciatica' – can cause pain in the calf.

Treatment See 'Back pain' section (p. 24).

Varicose veins These are explained in the 'Ankle swelling' section (p. 20). They can sometimes cause a mild ache in the calf, or when inflamed, areas of tenderness ('phlebitis').

Treatment This is discussed in the 'Ankle swelling' section

(p. 20). Phlebitis is treated with a couple of days' rest, a support stocking, and anti-inflammatories like aspirin or ibuprofen (available from the chemist).

Achilles tendon tear The Achilles tendon is the thick cord you can feel which attaches the lower end of your calf to your heel. A sudden stretch, especially going on tiptoe, can tear the tendon.

Treatment A suspected Achilles tendon tear needs urgent attention – go to casualty.

Deep vein thrombosis The arteries take blood to the leg muscles; the veins drain it back again. A clot – a liver-like lump – can form in one of these large veins. It's usually linked to being immobile – for example, being in a plaster because of a broken leg – or to pregnancy (or the few weeks after childbirth). It's also a bit more common in women who use the Pill, especially if they smoke.

Treatment Check it urgently with your GP: if she thinks you have a thrombosis it'll mean a trip to the hospital for blood-thinning tablets to dissolve the clot. Women who have had a deep vein thrombosis should no longer use the Pill for family planning, as this raises the chances of another one occurring.

Vascular disease Blood vessels (arteries) carry blood into the legs to supply the muscles with oxygen. If the arteries get furred up, the muscles can suffer from a lack of blood, especially during exercise. They complain by causing pain.

Treatment Stop smoking, keep exercising, and take half a soluble aspirin a day – all of these measures help to unblock the arteries. But it's worth seeing your GP, as you will need to see a specialist for further tests and treatment.

Neuropathy This is a disease of the nerves supplying sensation to the legs. It can be caused by a whole variety of problems, most of which are pretty rare. The two commonest culprits are diabetes and excessive alcohol: the high blood sugar and the alcohol, respectively, poison the nerves.

Treatment If alcohol is the cause, you've obviously got to stop as you have a serious problem and are probably an alcoholic. If you're having trouble stopping, or you think there might be some other cause – or you're known to be diabetic and you're wondering if you've developed neuropathy – see your GP.

Chest pain

N.B. If you have breast pain rather than chest pain, see 'Breast pain', p.40

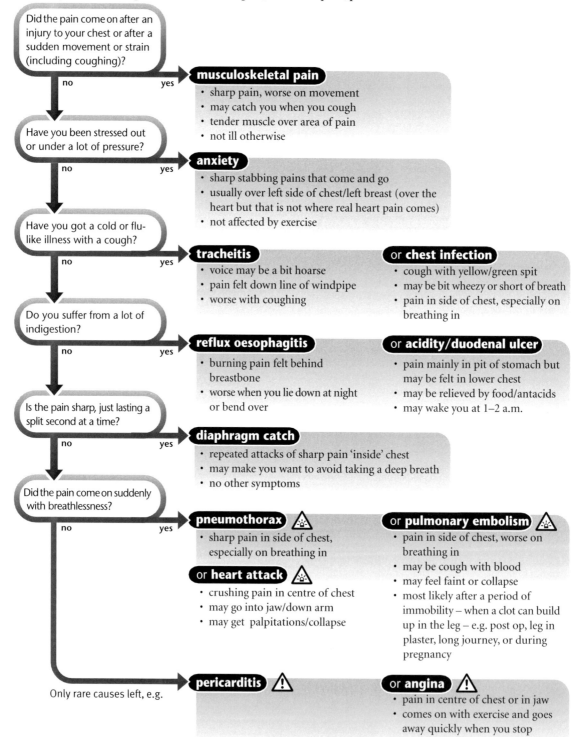

Did the pain come on after an injury to your chest or after a sudden movement or strain (including coughing)?

no → yes

musculoskeletal pain
- sharp pain, worse on movement
- may catch you when you cough
- tender muscle over area of pain
- not ill otherwise

Have you been stressed out or under a lot of pressure?

no → yes

anxiety
- sharp stabbing pains that come and go
- usually over left side of chest/left breast (over the heart but that is not where real heart pain comes)
- not affected by exercise

Have you got a cold or flu-like illness with a cough?

no → yes

tracheitis
- voice may be a bit hoarse
- pain felt down line of windpipe
- worse with coughing

or **chest infection**
- cough with yellow/green spit
- may be bit wheezy or short of breath
- pain in side of chest, especially on breathing in

Do you suffer from a lot of indigestion?

no → yes

reflux oesophagitis
- burning pain felt behind breastbone
- worse when you lie down at night or bend over

or **acidity/duodenal ulcer**
- pain mainly in pit of stomach but may be felt in lower chest
- may be relieved by food/antacids
- may wake you at 1–2 a.m.

Is the pain sharp, just lasting a split second at a time?

no → yes

diaphragm catch
- repeated attacks of sharp pain 'inside' chest
- may make you want to avoid taking a deep breath
- no other symptoms

Did the pain come on suddenly with breathlessness?

no → yes

pneumothorax
- sharp pain in side of chest, especially on breathing in

or **heart attack**
- crushing pain in centre of chest
- may go into jaw/down arm
- may get palpitations/collapse

or **pulmonary embolism**
- pain in side of chest, worse on breathing in
- may be cough with blood
- may feel faint or collapse
- most likely after a period of immobility – when a clot can build up in the leg – e.g. post op, leg in plaster, long journey, or during pregnancy

Only rare causes left, e.g.

pericarditis

or **angina**
- pain in centre of chest or in jaw
- comes on with exercise and goes away quickly when you stop

Musculoskeletal pain The muscle and bone which make up the rib cage can be inflamed by a muscle strain, a knock, or a virus.

Treatment This will settle down on its own, but can take up to a few weeks because the rib cage is very sensitive and is in constant 'use' (expanding and contracting with every breath you take). Painkillers or anti-inflammatories (such as ibuprofen) from the chemist will help, as will heat treatment (like a heat lamp or a hot water bottle).

Anxiety Feeling uptight tenses the muscles in the rib cage, which can cause various types of pains. If you're already anxious and you start getting chest pains, you're likely to worry that you've got something serious wrong, such as heart trouble. This creates more anxiety and worsening pains, and so a vicious cycle develops.

Treatment The key thing is to accept there's nothing seriously wrong as this will help you relax, easing the muscle tension. If you have trouble convincing yourself, discuss the situation with your GP. Also, try to sort out whatever is making you uptight in the first place; relaxation exercises and physical exercise will help too. For further details, see the 'Feeling tense' section (p. 64).

Tracheitis If you have a cold or the flu, the germ can go down your windpipe (the 'trachea'), causing tracheitis.

Treatment Antibiotics don't help. It'll go away on its own in a few days – in the meantime, try painkillers and steam inhalations, and avoid cigarette smoke.

Reflux oesophagitis This is explained, and the treatment outlined, in the 'Indigestion' section (p. 78). If the acid makes the gullet very sore, it can cause a pain felt in the chest.

Diaphragm catch The diaphragm is the internal sheet of muscle separating your chest from your guts. Diaphragm catch is thought to be an irritation of this muscle, although no one knows what causes it – but it's definitely harmless.

Treatment As the cause isn't known, there's nothing that you can really do to prevent it. It comes on and disappears so quickly it's not even worth taking a painkiller, as the pain will go long before any tablet has a chance to work. So just try to ignore it.

Acidity/duodenal ulcer This is explained, and the treatment discussed, in the 'Abdominal pain – recurrent' section (p. 10). Sometimes the pain is felt in the chest rather than the abdomen.

Chest infection A severe type of chest infection – pneumonia – can cause 'pleurisy'. This is explained further in the 'Cough' section (p. 46).

Angina or heart attack If the blood vessels which feed your heart get furred up, blood can have trouble getting through. As a result, the heart muscle gets starved of oxygen and complains by producing a tight pain across the chest, particularly when you're exerting yourself – this is 'angina'. If a blood vessel blocks totally, then the bit of heart muscle it supplies dies – this causes a sudden and severe pain across the chest (a heart attack or 'myocardial infarction'). The risk of angina or a heart attack is raised if you smoke, have heart disease in the family, are overweight, eat an unhealthy diet, have a high cholesterol level (a type of fat in the blood), have high blood pressure, or do little exercise – and particularly if you have any combination of these. But overall, these problems are very unlikely in women who've not reached the menopause.

Treatment If you think you're getting angina, you must see your GP. She'll probably start you on some medication; she'll also refer you to a heart specialist for further tests to confirm that this is the problem and to see if you need any other types of treatment. It's very important to sort out your lifestyle: your GP will give you advice about diet, weight loss, and exercise, and you'll need to pack in the cigarettes. If you think you might be having a heart attack, don't delay – call an ambulance straight away. The hospital doctors can give you treatment to ease the pain and protect your heart, but this has to be done as soon as possible. And while you're waiting for the paramedics, chew an aspirin, because this thins the blood and helps unblock the blood vessels.

Pericarditis This is an inflammation of the lining of the heart, which is usually caused by a virus.

Treatment You'll need to see your GP, who may well send you to hospital if she thinks you've got pericarditis.

Pneumothorax and pulmonary embolism
These are explained in the 'Shortness of breath' (p. 132) and 'Blood in spit' (p. 34) sections.

Cough

Do you have a cold or a sore throat?

no / yes

upper respiratory tract infection

- sneezing, runny nose, sore neck glands

or chest infection

- may develop after you have had a cold for a few days
- cough increases with some shortness of breath
- yellow/green spit
- may be wheezy
- may get chest pain, especially on breathing in

or asthma

- may be brought on by a cold

Is your cough mainly at night and/or worse after exercise?

no / yes

asthma

- cough is first symptom, wheeze if worsens
- history of being a 'chesty' child
- chest may feel 'tight', especially first thing in the morning

Is your cough mainly first thing in the morning or after a cigarette?

no / yes

smoker's cough if you cough/ spit first thing most mornings then you are at risk of developing chronic bronchitis or emphysema

or asthma see above

Are you on any regular medication, e.g. for high blood pressure?

no / yes

medication side-effect

e.g. from ACE inhibitors

Do you suffer from a lot of heartburn?

no / yes

acid reflux

- burning feeling behind breastbone
- worse when you lie down at night
- worse when you bend over

Only rare causes left, e.g.

tuberculosis ⚠️

or cancer of the lung ⚠️

Remember: ⚠️ means see your GP sharpish; ⚠️ means an urgent hospital job

Cough

NB In every case, smoking will aggravate the problem and may, if continued, make it more likely to come back again in the future. So we'll say it only once to avoid repetition: cut down – or better still, stop – smoking. More detail is provided in the 'Shortness of breath' section (p. 132).

Upper respiratory tract infection   The upper respiratory tract includes the ear, nose, throat, and windpipe. Infections are usually caused by viruses, the commonest resulting in the humble cold.

Treatment Paracetamol and a high fluid intake will ease the aches and pains and sore throat. Inhaling steam from a bowl of hot water, with a towel over your head (add menthol if you like) and propping yourself up at night will help the cough, whereas cough mixtures probably don't achieve a lot. The cough does have a purpose – it's the body's way of getting the germ out of your windpipe – so it's not surprising that it can take a week or two to go. And if the cold leaves you with lots of catarrh, this can drip down the back of the throat, especially at night, making the cough drag on. Again, inhalations may help. Don't bother your GP with this problem, though, because there's really nothing to do other than give it time to settle.

Chest infection   There are various types, the most likely being bronchitis. This is a complication of an upper respiratory tract infection (see above) in which the germ gets into the lungs. But if you're really ill, you might have pneumonia – a severe form of chest infection which can spread to the lining of the lung causing 'pleurisy'. This is more likely to be a complication of flu or chickenpox rather than a simple cold.

Treatment If your cough is showing no signs of settling after a few days with the treatment described for upper respiratory tract infection, or if you feel really rough or are having any trouble breathing, then it's worth seeing your GP – you may need antibiotics to clear the germ. And if it turns out you have pneumonia, you might even need to be admitted to hospital.

Smoker's cough   Cigarette smoke irritates the lungs, causing a cough. It also makes the lungs produce more protective mucus, which builds up as catarrh – this can only be shifted by coughing, and is often noticed more first thing in the morning. Remember that you don't necessarily have to be a smoker to develop a smoker's cough – breathing in other people's smoke (passive smoking) can cause it too.

Treatment See the 'Smoking' part of the 'Shortness of breath' section (p. 132).

Asthma   If the small airways in the lung narrow at times and clog up with phlegm, the result is a cough, wheezing, and shortness of breath. This is asthma. The exact cause is unknown but it can run in families, is linked to hay fever and eczema, and can be triggered by certain things, such as colds, pollen, changes in air temperature, stress, and exercise.

Treatment See your GP. You're likely to be prescribed treatment in the form of inhalers, which should sort out the problem, provided you use them as directed. There's not much you can do to prevent attacks unless there's obviously something that brings it on and which you can avoid (such as an allergy to cats). It's a sensible idea to keep in shape – swimming is thought to be particularly good exercise for asthmatics. If you're coughing a lot and are really tight-chested – or you're known to have asthma and you think your coughing is caused by a bad attack – then see your GP urgently as you may need some other treatment such as steroid tablets.

Medication side-effect   One group of treatments often prescribed for blood pressure problems – 'ACE inhibitors' – have cough as their main side-effect.

Treatment Discuss the situation with your GP. You'll either need to put up with the cough – if it isn't too troublesome – or be switched to a different type of blood pressure pill.

Acid reflux   If the valve at the top of your stomach doesn't work properly, the acid in your stomach can leak up into your gullet – this is acid reflux. When you lie down it can spill right up into the throat, causing spasms of coughing.

Treatment Go on a sensible diet if you're overweight, don't eat too late at night, and try an antacid from the chemist. Also, raise the head of your bed a couple of inches with blocks – gravity will then keep the acid in your stomach when you're asleep.

Rare medical causes   There is a whole heap of very unusual causes. Cancer is rare in the under 45s, and incredibly unlikely in non-smokers. Other possibilities include TB and rare lung diseases. You're unlikely to need to worry about any of these.

Treatment See your GP. If she's concerned, she'll arrange the necessary tests.

Deafness

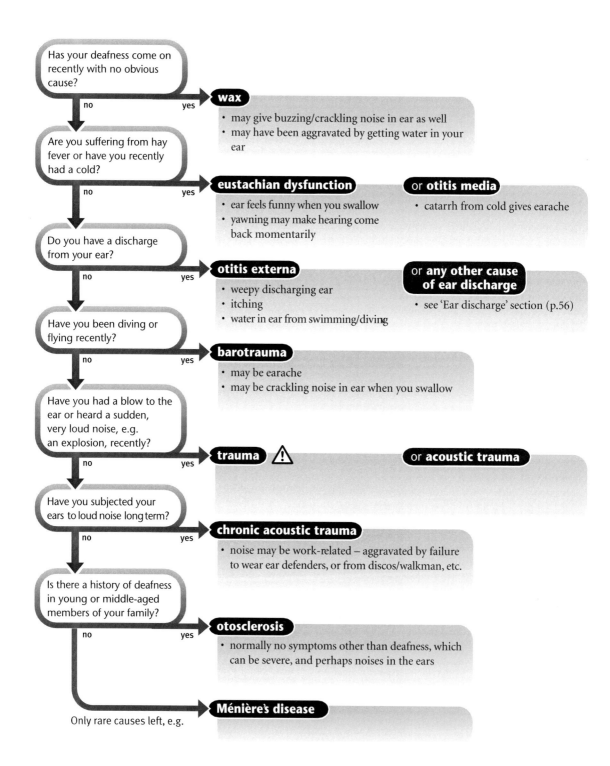

Has your deafness come on recently with no obvious cause?

wax
- may give buzzing/crackling noise in ear as well
- may have been aggravated by getting water in your ear

Are you suffering from hay fever or have you recently had a cold?

eustachian dysfunction
- ear feels funny when you swallow
- yawning may make hearing come back momentarily

or otitis media
- catarrh from cold gives earache

Do you have a discharge from your ear?

otitis externa
- weepy discharging ear
- itching
- water in ear from swimming/diving

or any other cause of ear discharge
- see 'Ear discharge' section (p.56)

Have you been diving or flying recently?

barotrauma
- may be earache
- may be crackling noise in ear when you swallow

Have you had a blow to the ear or heard a sudden, very loud noise, e.g. an explosion, recently?

trauma ⚠

or acoustic trauma

Have you subjected your ears to loud noise long term?

chronic acoustic trauma
- noise may be work-related – aggravated by failure to wear ear defenders, or from discos/walkman, etc.

Is there a history of deafness in young or middle-aged members of your family?

otosclerosis
- normally no symptoms other than deafness, which can be severe, and perhaps noises in the ears

Ménière's disease

Only rare causes left, e.g.

Ear wax The ear canal (the tube you can put your little finger into and which leads to your ear drum) produces wax. This is quite normal, but if a lot of wax builds up – or it becomes wedged down inside the canal because you've been ramming cotton buds in your ear – it can block the ear canal completely, causing deafness.

Treatment Don't try to gouge the wax out yourself. Cotton buds will just push it down further and harden it, making it more difficult to shift. Instead, soften the wax for a couple of days using ear drops from the chemist. This may solve the problem. If it doesn't, see your GP or practice nurse, who will probably syringe the wax out for you.

Eustachian tube dysfunction The eustachian tube is the internal tube which connects the inner part of the ear to the back of the throat. Its job is to equalize pressure changes and drain catarrh from the ear. When it gets blocked – most commonly because of a cold or hay fever – it doesn't work properly (eustachian tube dysfunction), causing a build-up of catarrh which results in deafness.

Treatment Usually, the problem sorts itself out on its own within a few days. Inhaling steam from a bowl of hot water, with some added menthol, may help by shifting some of the catarrh. If it drags on for a while, a technique called the Valsalva manoeuvre is worth trying. The trick is to build up air pressure in your mouth and throat – this can open up the eustachian tube. The easiest way to do this is to simply blow up a balloon. You may need to keep trying this for some days – eventually, the ear should start to crackle or pop, and the deafness will clear. If the cause might be hay fever, try one of the over-the-counter anti-hay fever nose sprays, as this is likely to solve the problem.

Otitis media This is explained in the 'Earache' section (p. 54). The infection inflames the drum, causing deafness.

Treatment See the 'Earache' section (p. 54). The deafness is usually the last symptom to settle – it may take a few weeks before your hearing seems completely normal again.

Any cause of ear discharge Various problems – particularly infections – can cause a discharge from the ear (see the 'Ear discharge' section, p. 56). If the discharge blocks the ear canal, then your hearing is bound to be affected.

Treatment See the 'Ear discharge' section (p. 56).

Barotrauma This is the term used to describe problems caused by outside pressure changes affecting the ear. The most common causes are air travel and scuba diving – the deafness results from a build-up of fluid deep inside the ear and is especially likely if these activities are done when you have a cold.

Treatment The problem will correct itself, but it can take many weeks. The tricks described under eustachian tube dysfunction (above) may help.

Acoustic trauma This is explained in the section on 'Noises in the ear' (p. 106).

Treatment There is no magic cure. Discuss the situation with your GP if it is becoming a problem – she may refer you to an Ear, Nose, and Throat ('ENT') specialist to consider a hearing aid.

Otosclerosis The inside of the ear contains tiny bones which move to amplify the sound. These bones can sometimes stiffen up and not move as they should, causing deafness which slowly gets worse – this is otosclerosis. This problem can run in families.

Treatment You will need to see an ENT specialist to confirm this diagnosis. If necessary, it can be treated with surgery.

Trauma This is explained, and the treatment outlined, in the 'Earache' section (p. 54).

Ménière's disease This is a disease caused by an increase in the pressure of the fluid which circulates in the deepest, most complex parts of the ear. This high pressure affects the hearing and balance apparatus, resulting in deafness, dizziness, and ringing in the ears. Quite why it should happen remains unclear.

Treatment See your GP – it's likely that you'll be referred to an ENT specialist to be checked out.

Other rare causes These include small-print diseases such as unusual viruses, types of stroke, and growths on the nerve of the ear.

Treatment Discuss the problem with your GP, who will arrange any necessary tests or hospital appointments.

Diarrhoea

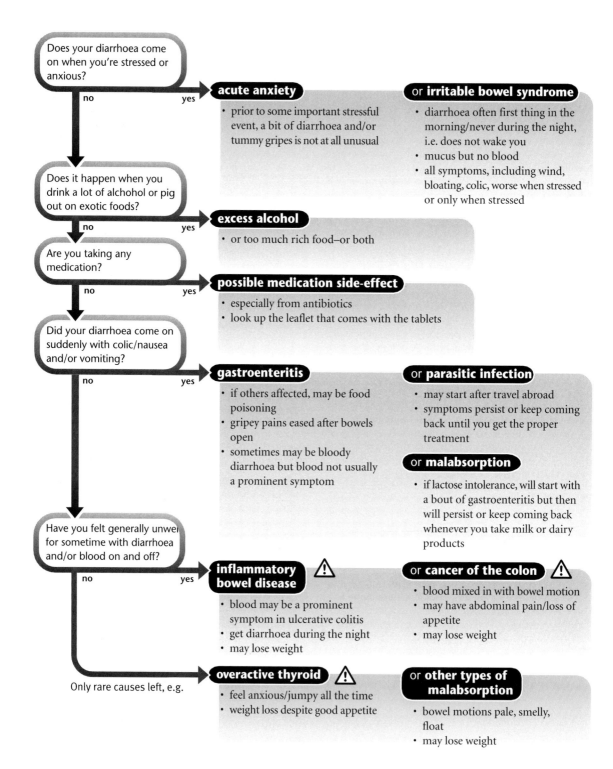

Does your diarrhoea come on when you're stressed or anxious?

no / yes

acute anxiety
- prior to some important stressful event, a bit of diarrhoea and/or tummy gripes is not at all unusual

or **irritable bowel syndrome**
- diarrhoea often first thing in the morning/never during the night, i.e. does not wake you
- mucus but no blood
- all symptoms, including wind, bloating, colic, worse when stressed or only when stressed

Does it happen when you drink a lot of alchohol or pig out on exotic foods?

no / yes

excess alcohol
- or too much rich food—or both

Are you taking any medication?

no / yes

possible medication side-effect
- especially from antibiotics
- look up the leaflet that comes with the tablets

Did your diarrhoea come on suddenly with colic/nausea and/or vomiting?

no / yes

gastroenteritis
- if others affected, may be food poisoning
- gripey pains eased after bowels open
- sometimes may be bloody diarrhoea but blood not usually a prominent symptom

or **parasitic infection**
- may start after travel abroad
- symptoms persist or keep coming back until you get the proper treatment

or **malabsorption**
- if lactose intolerance, will start with a bout of gastroenteritis but then will persist or keep coming back whenever you take milk or dairy products

Have you felt generally unwell for sometime with diarrhoea and/or blood on and off?

no / yes

inflammatory bowel disease ⚠
- blood may be a prominent symptom in ulcerative colitis
- get diarrhoea during the night
- may lose weight

or **cancer of the colon** ⚠
- blood mixed in with bowel motion
- may have abdominal pain/loss of appetite
- may lose weight

Only rare causes left, e.g.

overactive thyroid ⚠
- feel anxious/jumpy all the time
- weight loss despite good appetite

or **other types of malabsorption**
- bowel motions pale, smelly, float
- may lose weight

Acute anxiety Important life events such as exams, driving tests, weddings, court appearances, and so on can make your bowel overactive – especially first thing in the morning when you get up.
Treatment This is totally normal, so no treatment is needed.

Gastroenteritis A germ in the bowel, usually through something you've eaten – hence the term 'food poisoning'.
Treatment This is covered in the 'Abdominal pain – one-off' section (p. 8).

Irritable bowel syndrome (IBS) The bowel is simply a long muscular tube. When 'irritable', it squeezes too much, too little, or in an uncoordinated way, resulting in the typical symptoms of IBS.
Treatment Most of the treatment is covered in the 'Abdominal pain – recurrent' section (p. 10). When diarrhoea is the main symptom, an over-the-counter medicine, such as loperamide, may help, although medicines like this are probably best kept to a minimum. Cutting down your fibre intake may also help – but could cause problems too if you also get constipated at times with your IBS.

Excess alcohol Drinking too much – especially binge drinking – often results in diarrhoea. The sheer volume of fluid may be the cause, or it might be that you have mild irritable bowel syndrome, which is aggravated by alcohol.
Treatment Cut down on the alcohol – and avoid binges.

Medication side-effect Just about any medication – prescribed or bought over the counter – can cause diarrhoea. The worst culprits are probably antibiotics and anti-inflammatory drugs like ibuprofen.
Treatment Try to grin and bear it if the treatment is just a short course, such as a few days of antibiotics for an infection. If that seems impossible, seek an alternative medicine: your pharmacist or GP will be able to help you. If the diarrhoea seems to be a side-effect of long-term medication prescribed by your doctor, you'll need to discuss the situation with her. You may be advised to try without the treatment, or you might be prescribed something else instead.

Malabsorption Some diseases of the gut stop your food being broken down (i.e. digested) or taken into the body (i.e. absorbed) properly. This leads to diarrhoea, and is known as malabsorption. Two of the commonest causes are coeliac disease, in which you cannot absorb gluten (found in wheat, rye, barley, and oats), and lactose intolerance, in which you cannot tolerate lactose (a sugar found in milk).
Treatment You will need to see your GP. She'll look into it either by arranging special tests or by sending you to a dietitian who, by cutting out certain items in your diet, will be able to work out what the precise problem is. The dietitian is obviously helpful in treatment too, as the cure often lies in knowing which foods to avoid. Other types of malabsorption may need specialist treatment.

Parasitic infections Some unusual infections of the gut are caused by parasites (organisms which live off other organisms). These microscopic creatures live in the wall of the bowel, causing, amongst other symptoms, diarrhoea. They are usually – but not always – picked up from travel abroad.
Treatment If you think you may have this type of problem, see your GP. You'll need tests and, if they confirm the diagnosis, a course of antibiotics.

Inflammatory bowel disease Crohn's disease and ulcerative colitis are the 'inflammatory bowel diseases' – illnesses which inflame the lining of the gut, causing diarrhoea which may be bloody, often with other symptoms like weight loss. The precise cause remains a mystery.
Treatment See your GP. She will arrange tests, which will usually include seeing a bowel specialist in hospital. Your treatment will depend on the type of disease you have, and its pattern, and may involve tablets – sometimes lifelong – and enemas (liquids squirted up into the bottom).

Overactive thyroid The thyroid gland sits in the middle of the front of the neck. It produces thyroid hormone, which controls the body's activity. If too much is produced – 'hyperthyroidism' – one of the effects is persistent diarrhoea.
Treatment This is covered in the 'Excess sweating' section (p. 58).

Colon cancer The colon is the large bowel – the last part of your gut which ends up at the rectum and anus (back passage). Colon cancer is rare in the under 40s. However, there is some increase in risk if you have had polyps (small benign growths) of the colon – or they run in your family – or you've had severe ulcerative colitis for years.
Treatment See your GP, who will arrange the necessary tests and an appointment with a specialist.

Dizziness

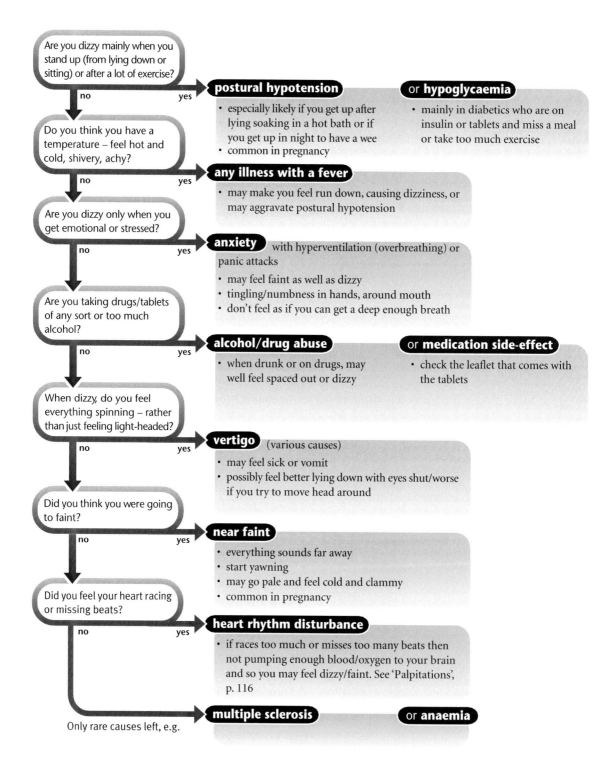

Are you dizzy mainly when you stand up (from lying down or sitting) or after a lot of exercise? — no / yes

postural hypotension
- especially likely if you get up after lying soaking in a hot bath or if you get up in night to have a wee
- common in pregnancy

or hypoglycaemia
- mainly in diabetics who are on insulin or tablets and miss a meal or take too much exercise

Do you think you have a temperature – feel hot and cold, shivery, achy? — no / yes

any illness with a fever
- may make you feel run down, causing dizziness, or may aggravate postural hypotension

Are you dizzy only when you get emotional or stressed? — no / yes

anxiety with hyperventilation (overbreathing) or panic attacks
- may feel faint as well as dizzy
- tingling/numbness in hands, around mouth
- don't feel as if you can get a deep enough breath

Are you taking drugs/tablets of any sort or too much alcohol? — no / yes

alcohol/drug abuse
- when drunk or on drugs, may well feel spaced out or dizzy

or medication side-effect
- check the leaflet that comes with the tablets

When dizzy, do you feel everything spinning – rather than just feeling light-headed? — no / yes

vertigo (various causes)
- may feel sick or vomit
- possibly feel better lying down with eyes shut/worse if you try to move head around

Did you think you were going to faint? — no / yes

near faint
- everything sounds far away
- start yawning
- may go pale and feel cold and clammy
- common in pregnancy

Did you feel your heart racing or missing beats? — no / yes

heart rhythm disturbance
- if races too much or misses too many beats then not pumping enough blood/oxygen to your brain and so you may feel dizzy/faint. See 'Palpitations', p. 116

multiple sclerosis **or anaemia**

Only rare causes left, e.g.

Postural hypotension If you stand up suddenly, your blood pressure can drop. Momentarily, not enough blood gets through to the brain, which is starved of oxygen for a few seconds. The result is light-headedness, which quickly passes off. A typical example is when you leap out of a hot bath to answer the 'phone. This problem is also more common when you're pregnant.

Treatment This type of dizziness is almost always normal, although it can be made worse by some prescribed treatments (such as blood pressure pills and antidepressants). Talk to your GP if you think that your treatment is causing you a problem.

Any illness with a high temperature Feeling a bit light-headed – especially on standing – is a common symptom whenever you've got a virus or some other infection (e.g. flu, a tummy bug, tonsillitis, or a chest infection).

Treatment The dizziness itself doesn't need treatment as it's simply part of the overall grotty feeling. Use your main symptom (such as cough and sore throat) to guide you to the right section of this book.

Anxiety Being uptight can make you feel dizzy, especially if it leads to hyperventilation or panic attacks. See the 'Feeling tense' (p. 64) or 'Shortness of breath' (p. 132) sections for further details and advice about treatment.

Near faint A near faint is simply a faint that you just about manage to prevent – see the 'Loss of consciousness' section (p. 88) for more details. Faints and near faints are more common in early pregnancy because the hormones tend to lower your blood pressure.

Alcohol/drug abuse It's hardly surprising that you'll feel dizzy when the aim is to get out of your head.

Treatment The dizziness itself isn't harmful, unless of course you keel over and injure yourself. But drug and alcohol abuse obviously can be. If you think you have a problem and you want help, see your GP or contact the local drug or alcohol unit.

Vertigo This is the medical word to describe an unpleasant 'head spinning' feeling (like when you've just stepped off a carousel). It's caused by something going wrong with your balance mechanism, and there are lots of different causes.

The most common are viral labyrinthitis (a germ affecting the ear, usually with a cold) and benign positional vertigo (vertigo which keeps coming on whenever you turn your head in certain positions). An alcohol binge can have a very similar effect.

Treatment This depends on the cause, so you'll need to speak to your GP. The viral type goes away on its own, usually after a few days. Benign positional vertigo may need the help of an Ear, Nose, and Throat ('ENT') specialist. And remember not to drive until you can turn your head without the world spinning round.

Medication side-effect Some prescribed treatments can cause light-headedness. They can also lead to postural hypotension (see above).

Treatment Take a look at the leaflet in the pack. If it mentions dizziness, have a word with your GP – she may be able to stop the treatment or prescribe something else instead.

Hypoglycaemia This means a low blood sugar level. The sugar in your blood fuels the brain – so if the levels drop, maybe because you've missed a meal or you've done an unusual amount of exercise, you tend to feel a bit light-headed. This is particularly common in diabetics on treatment (the pills or injections lower the blood sugar).

Treatment Eat regularly and, in particular, don't skip breakfast. If you're a diabetic, check out the 'Hypoglycaemia' part of the 'Loss of consciousness' section (p. 88).

Heart rhythm disturbance If your heart beats too slowly, too quickly, or erratically, it may not pump enough blood through to the brain, causing dizziness – see the 'Palpitations' section, p. 116 (especially the 'Supraventricular tachycardia' part), for more details.

Rare medical problems A whole load of small-print problems (including anaemia, multiple sclerosis, kidney failure, and heart valve problems) can cause dizziness, but you're highly unlikely to have any of them – and they tend to cause lots of other symptoms which give the game away.

Treatment If you think you might be suffering one of these rarities, you're probably wrong, but have a word with your GP.

Earache

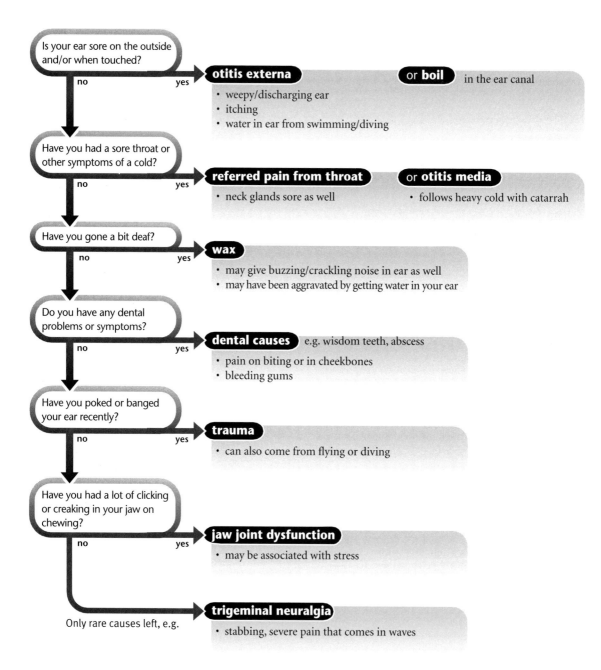

Is your ear sore on the outside and/or when touched?

no / yes

otitis externa or **boil** in the ear canal
- weepy/discharging ear
- itching
- water in ear from swimming/diving

Have you had a sore throat or other symptoms of a cold?

no / yes

referred pain from throat or **otitis media**
- neck glands sore as well
- follows heavy cold with catarrah

Have you gone a bit deaf?

no / yes

wax
- may give buzzing/crackling noise in ear as well
- may have been aggravated by getting water in your ear

Do you have any dental problems or symptoms?

no / yes

dental causes e.g. wisdom teeth, abscess
- pain on biting or in cheekbones
- bleeding gums

Have you poked or banged your ear recently?

no / yes

trauma
- can also come from flying or diving

Have you had a lot of clicking or creaking in your jaw on chewing?

no / yes

jaw joint dysfunction
- may be associated with stress

Only rare causes left, e.g.

trigeminal neuralgia
- stabbing, severe pain that comes in waves

Earache

Otitis externa An infection of the outer ear canal – the bit you can get your finger into.

Treatment If you keep water out of your ears and stop prodding about with cotton buds, then it may settle down on its own. Ban buds and water anyway in the long run to stop repeated attacks: the ear canal can clean itself without your help, and waterlogging can be avoided by using ear plugs (e.g. cotton wool dipped in vaseline) when washing your hair or swimming. For a bad attack, you'll need drops or a spray from your GP. And if you get eczema of the ear canal, hydrocortisone 1% cream from the chemist may help.

Boil This is just like a boil anywhere else – an infection of the skin which can develop into a pus-filled lump. Except that, being in the confined space of the ear canal, it hurts like hell.

Treatment Painkillers and cross your fingers – it's likely to go by itself in a few days but, if it's getting worse, your GP may prescribe antibiotics.

Wax Most people react to wax by attacking their ears with cotton buds. This makes matters worse as the wax simply gets wedged further in so that it presses on the ear drum, causing pain.

Treatment First, throw those buds away. Next, use drops from the chemist to soften the wax. This may solve the problem, but if it just makes you deafer, see the practice nurse who will syringe it for you.

Otitis media An infection of the eardrum, usually with a cold. It's the commonest cause of earache in children.

Treatment Try some painkillers from the chemist for 24 hours. If it's showing no signs of improving, contact your GP, as you may need antibiotics.

Referred pain Problems in a variety of other areas can 'send' the pain to the ear. For example, throat infections and wear and tear of the bones in the neck can result in pain which feels as though it comes from the ear.

Treatment Figure out where it's coming from, look up the appropriate section in this book and, hey presto, problem solved.

Dental causes All sorts of dental problems, such as wisdom tooth trouble or abscesses, can result in earache.

Treatment Bite the bullet and see a dentist.

Trauma Assaulting your ear runs the risk of causing damage – probably just a scrape to the canal, though you can seriously damage the eardrum if you're really determined. A loud noise or a smack to the side of the head (which includes a badly executed dive into a swimming pool) can also cause painful damage. Pressure changes – called 'barotrauma' – which you might feel when flying or scuba diving can also cause earache.

Treatment Sudden pain after trauma, especially with deafness, is not good news – you may have done some significant damage. See your doctor asap or go to casualty. The ache caused by barotrauma usually settles down quickly, although your hearing may feel a bit muffled for a week or two.

Jaw joint dysfunction A problem of the hinge joint between the jaw and the skull – there's one on each side, right next to each ear. If your bite is slightly out of line, or you grind your teeth out of habit or when tense, the joint can get inflamed and painful.

Treatment Use painkillers for a bad attack, but to get it cured you probably need to see your dentist.

Trigeminal neuralgia Neuralgia is a sharp pain coming from a nerve – in this case, the 'trigeminal', which supplies the sensation to the ear.

Treatment Wait and see. It'll probably fizzle out on its own after a while. If not, discuss the situation with your doctor.

Ear discharge

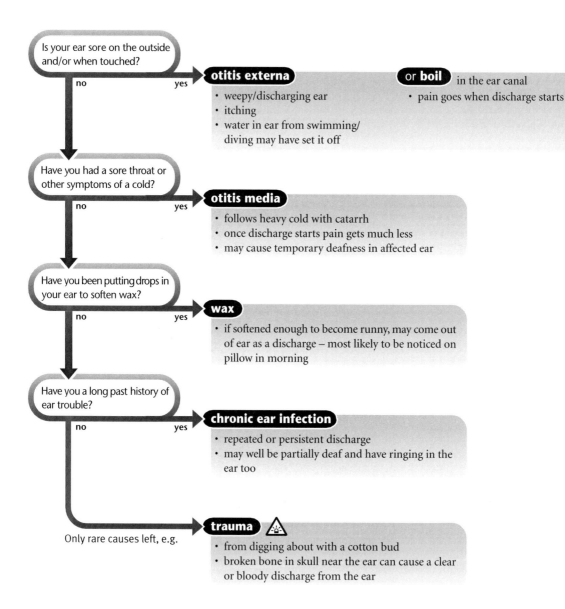

Is your ear sore on the outside and/or when touched?

no → yes →

otitis externa
- weepy/discharging ear
- itching
- water in ear from swimming/ diving may have set it off

or boil in the ear canal
- pain goes when discharge starts

Have you had a sore throat or other symptoms of a cold?

no → yes →

otitis media
- follows heavy cold with catarrh
- once discharge starts pain gets much less
- may cause temporary deafness in affected ear

Have you been putting drops in your ear to soften wax?

no → yes →

wax
- if softened enough to become runny, may come out of ear as a discharge – most likely to be noticed on pillow in morning

Have you a long past history of ear trouble?

no → yes →

chronic ear infection
- repeated or persistent discharge
- may well be partially deaf and have ringing in the ear too

Only rare causes left, e.g.

trauma
- from digging about with a cotton bud
- broken bone in skull near the ear can cause a clear or bloody discharge from the ear

Remember: ⚠ means see your GP sharpish; ⚠ means an urgent hospital job

Otitis externa This is explained, and its treatment outlined, in the 'Earache' section (p. 54).

Boil This is an infection which produces a lump full of pus. This can happen in the ear canal where, because of the confined space, it'll hurt like hell. If you just grit your teeth, or load yourself with painkillers, you'll find either that the boil just disappears, or it bursts, leaking a discharge out of your ear.

Treatment By the time the boil is discharging, it's curing itself. The pain usually eases as soon as the discharge starts. The muck should disappear after a couple of days – if it doesn't, get your GP to take a look.

Otitis media This is an infection of the eardrum, usually with a cold. Pus can build up under pressure behind the eardrum, causing pain and, sometimes, a hole in the drum, so the pus escapes in the form of an ear discharge.

Treatment As the discharge starts, the pain usually eases up because the pressure on the eardrum is relieved. Unless the discharge and pain settle down quickly over a day or so, this type of infection requires antibiotics (in the form of medicine or drops) – so see your GP. The fact that your ear has discharged means that there must be a hole in your eardrum. This can take a few weeks to heal, so don't be surprised if your hearing seems dodgy for a while (and keep water out of your ears until everything seems back to normal). If the discharge keeps coming back, or your hearing isn't 100% again after a month, get your GP to take another look.

Wax It's normal to have wax in your ears. Some people seem to produce loads, others hardly any. If you have a build-up of wax, it can come out as a hard lump or as

runny, brown goo. The latter is particularly likely if you've been using ear drops, maybe because the excess wax was making you deaf.

Treatment As wax is normal, it doesn't need treatment. Clean up any wax you can see, but avoid the temptation to attack your ear canal (the bit you can get your little finger into) with cotton buds – this simply wedges the wax back in and can damage your eardrum.

Chronic ear infection Sometimes, an infection like otitis media fails to clear or keeps coming back. This is known as a chronic ear infection (the chronic refers to the fact that it carries on a long time, not that it is more painful than other types of ear infection). It usually means that the eardrum still has a hole in it which won't heal, and it can result in a lot of damage to your hearing apparatus.

Treatment Get it checked out by your GP; if she can't sort it out, she'll refer you to an Ear, Nose, and Throat ('ENT') specialist.

Trauma The most likely type of trauma involves you digging around with a cotton bud. This can graze the ear canal, causing a slight bleed. But if you're really determined, you can damage the eardrum, in which case you'll get pain, blood, and a sudden problem with your hearing. Another, less likely, type of trauma is a serious head injury causing a broken bone in the skull near your ear. This can result in the ear losing a bloody or clear discharge.

Treatment If it's just a graze, don't worry about it – it'll heal itself. Just avoid cotton buds in future. If you think you've done more serious damage, seek medical help asap. And if you've fractured a bone in your skull – you won't be reading this because you'll be in casualty.

Excess sweating

 If you are a diabetic on treatment, excess sweating may be a sign you are going 'hypo' (hypoglycaemic) – if in doubt, take sugar.

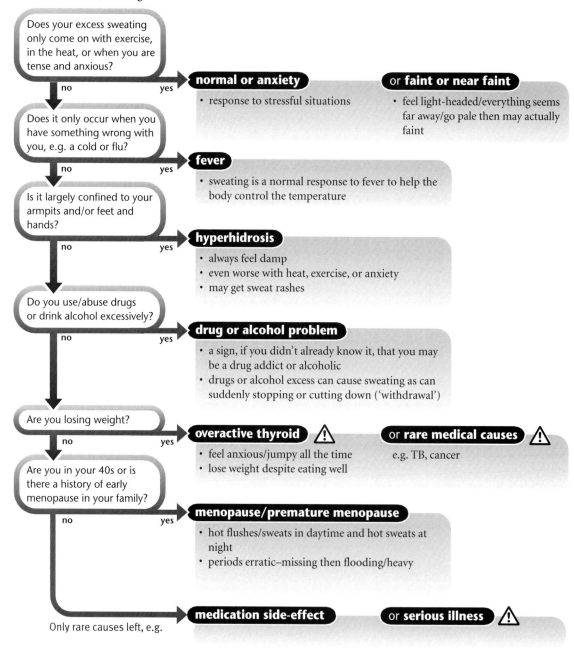

Does your excess sweating only come on with exercise, in the heat, or when you are tense and anxious?

no / yes

normal or anxiety
• response to stressful situations

or faint or near faint
• feel light-headed/everything seems far away/go pale then may actually faint

Does it only occur when you have something wrong with you, e.g. a cold or flu?

no / yes

fever
• sweating is a normal response to fever to help the body control the temperature

Is it largely confined to your armpits and/or feet and hands?

no / yes

hyperhidrosis
• always feel damp
• even worse with heat, exercise, or anxiety
• may get sweat rashes

Do you use/abuse drugs or drink alcohol excessively?

no / yes

drug or alcohol problem
• a sign, if you didn't already know it, that you may be a drug addict or alcoholic
• drugs or alcohol excess can cause sweating as can suddenly stopping or cutting down ('withdrawal')

Are you losing weight?

no / yes

overactive thyroid
• feel anxious/jumpy all the time
• lose weight despite eating well

or rare medical causes
e.g. TB, cancer

Are you in your 40s or is there a history of early menopause in your family?

no / yes

menopause/premature menopause
• hot flushes/sweats in daytime and hot sweats at night
• periods erratic–missing then flooding/heavy

Only rare causes left, e.g.

medication side-effect

or serious illness

'Normal' Everything about the human body varies between individuals. Sweating is no exception: some people simply sweat more than others. Being overweight tends to aggravate the problem.

Treatment Not a lot you can do about normality, other than common-sense measures to keep the problem to a minimum – such as keeping cool, wearing light, loosely fitting clothes, and finding an effective antiperspirant and, if necessary, losing weight.

Fever This is the body's response to an infection (usually a virus, such as flu). It pushes the temperature up to try to fight the germ off, and this causes sweating.

Treatment Regular paracetamol and plenty of cool fluids. The cause of the fever itself may need treating if it isn't a virus (see the 'High temperature' section, p. 74).

Anxiety It's obviously normal to feel anxious sometimes, in certain situations. In some people, this feeling is exaggerated, or stays most of the time. Sweating often accompanies anxiety of this sort.

Treatment This will depend on the cause of the anxiety (see 'Feeling tense' section, p. 64). In general, burning off nervous energy through increased physical exercise, and trying relaxation therapy (such as relaxation tapes), often help.

Faint or near faint Faints are explained, and their treatment outlined, in the 'Loss of consciousness' section (p. 88). If you're about to faint, you may find you suddenly start to sweat – this stops when the faint is over.

Hypoglycaemia This is also explained in the 'Loss of consciousness' section (p. 88). As in fainting, sweating accompanies the attack.

Menopause/premature menopause Excess sweating is one of the many symptoms the hormone changes of the menopause can cause. For further details, see the 'Flushing' section (p. 66).

Hyperhidrosis An over-production of sweat on the palms and soles and in the armpits. It is simply an extreme of 'normal' but can be a real nuisance.

Treatment Strong antiperspirant roll-ons containing aluminium hexahydrate are available from the chemist. These especially help the armpits, but do less for the palms and soles. They can also cause dryness or itching of the skin, but this can, in turn, be treated with hydrocortisone 1% cream, also available over the counter. If this fails and you're desperate, see your GP. There are some tablet treatments which can help, or she can refer you to a dermatologist for hospital-based treatment. Surgery is used as a last resort – this involves either removing the sweat-producing skin of the armpit or cutting the nerves which control the sweat glands in the palms.

Drug or alcohol abuse (or withdrawal) Drinking too much alcohol, or using illicit drugs such as amphetamines, can cause excess sweating. Stopping drugs (e.g. heroin) or alcohol suddenly leads to symptoms of withdrawal, when the body craves what it's missing. Sweating is a common sign of drug or alcohol withdrawal.

Treatment If you're having problems controlling the problem yourself, see your GP or local drug or alcohol advisory service for help.

Overactive thyroid The thyroid gland sits in the middle of the front of the neck. It produces thyroid hormone, which controls the body's activity – too little and you slow up, too much and you feel overactive. The latter is called hyperthyroidism, and this can result in excessive sweating.

Treatment A GP job, as it requires a blood test to confirm the diagnosis – then, usually, referral to a specialist for treatment.

Medication side-effect A few prescribed treatments, such as antidepressants, can cause sweating as a side-effect – although sweating may also be caused by the problem the drug is trying to treat, like depression and anxiety.

Treatment If your GP thinks your problem is a side-effect of a treatment you are taking, she may be able to stop the drug or prescribe an alternative.

Rare medical causes Very rarely, persistent bouts of sweating, especially at night, are caused by serious illness such as TB, certain types of arthritis, or cancers of the immune system.

Treatment Your GP will arrange any necessary tests.

Excessive hair

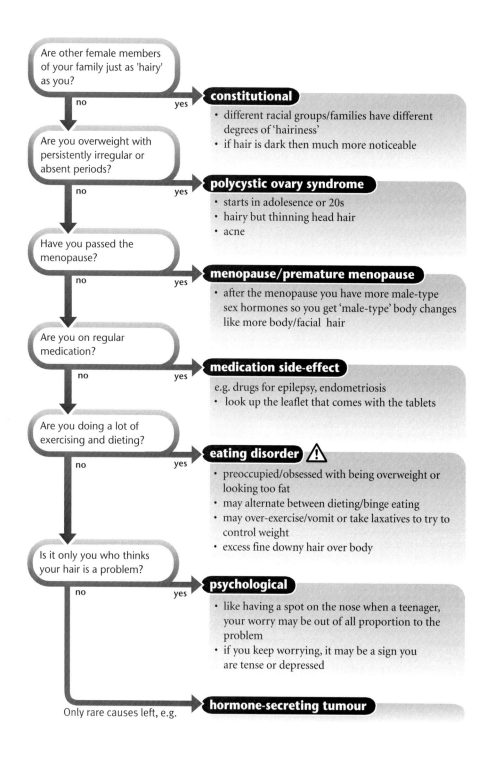

Are other female members of your family just as 'hairy' as you?

no / yes

constitutional
- different racial groups/families have different degrees of 'hairiness'
- if hair is dark then much more noticeable

Are you overweight with persistently irregular or absent periods?

no / yes

polycystic ovary syndrome
- starts in adolesence or 20s
- hairy but thinning head hair
- acne

Have you passed the menopause?

no / yes

menopause/premature menopause
- after the menopause you have more male-type sex hormones so you get 'male-type' body changes like more body/facial hair

Are you on regular medication?

no / yes

medication side-effect
e.g. drugs for epilepsy, endometriosis
- look up the leaflet that comes with the tablets

Are you doing a lot of exercising and dieting?

no / yes

eating disorder
- preoccupied/obsessed with being overweight or looking too fat
- may alternate between dieting/binge eating
- may over-exercise/vomit or take laxatives to try to control weight
- excess fine downy hair over body

Is it only you who thinks your hair is a problem?

no / yes

psychological
- like having a spot on the nose when a teenager, your worry may be out of all proportion to the problem
- if you keep worrying, it may be a sign you are tense or depressed

Only rare causes left, e.g.

hormone-secreting tumour

Constitutional Like everything else in life, hairiness varies between individuals. Often it's simply 'handed down', so other women in your family will have suffered the same problem. Or it may be linked with your race: women of Mediterranean, Middle Eastern, South Asian, or Afro-Caribbean origin tend to be 'hairier' than other women.

Treatment As this is quite normal, and not a sign of disease, no treatment is needed. But if you feel it's unsightly and would like to improve the situation, there are a number of cosmetic treatments which can help. These include plucking hairs (if only one or two areas are affected), depilatory creams (available from the chemist), bleaching, waxing, and shaving. Electrolysis can be very effective, but make sure you go somewhere reputable as there is a risk of scarring.

Polycystic ovary syndrome This is explained in the 'Absent periods' section (p. 18).

Treatment See the 'Absent periods' section (p. 18) for a general discussion about the treatment of this problem. Any of the suggestions mentioned above under 'Constitutional' may be used for polycystic ovary syndrome. If these don't help much then it's worth seeing your GP – there is a hormone treatment, which also acts as a contraceptive pill, which, given time, can ease the problem.

Menopause/premature menopause This is explained in the 'Flushing' section (p. 66). Excess hairiness is just one of the changes which your body might suffer after the menopause.

Treatment This is fully discussed in the 'Flushing' section (p. 66).

Medication side-effect A few prescribed treatments, such as some drugs for epilepsy and endometriosis, can cause excessive hairiness as a side-effect. Anabolic steroid abuse by athletes can result in the same problem.

Treatment Discuss the situation with your GP. If she agrees that this might be the problem, she may be able to stop the treatment or switch you to an alternative. If you need to continue with the same medication, you can always try the cosmetic measures described above. And if you're abusing anabolic steroids – stop.

Psychological Occasionally, the complaint of feeling excessively hairy is just a symptom of feeling generally unhappy about yourself, so that you notice things which are actually insignificant and which usually don't bother you. The underlying cause is usually tension or depression.

Treatment See the 'Feeling tense' section (p. 64) and the 'Depression' part of the 'Feeling down' section (p. 62).

Eating disorders Eating disorders like anorexia nervosa can cause hormone changes which affect hair growth – usually resulting in an excess of fine downy hair over most of the body.

Treatment See the 'Weight loss' section (p. 164).

Hormone-secreting tumour Very rarely, excess hair growth can be caused by a tumour which produces hormones. These tumours can occur in the ovaries or elsewhere.

Treatment It's highly unlikely that this type of illness will be the cause of your symptom – but if you're concerned, see your GP, who will arrange any necessary tests or, if concerned, will send you to a specialist.

Feeling down

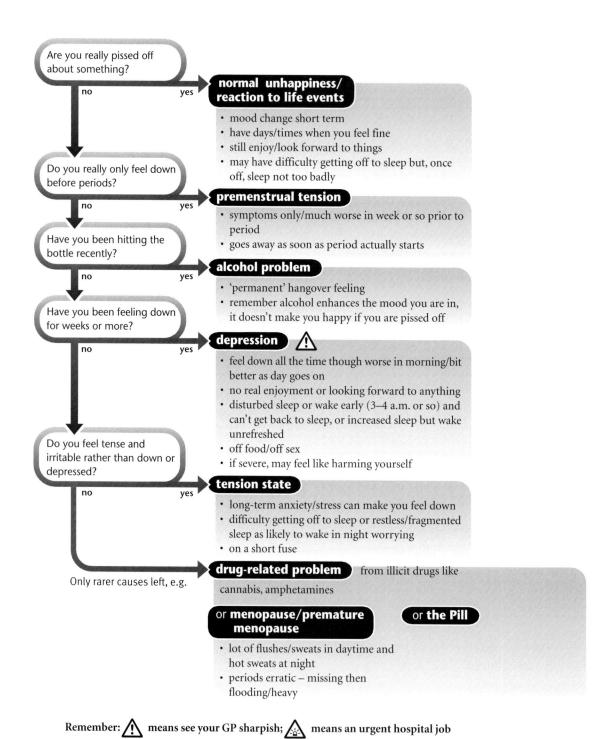

Are you really pissed off about something?
no → yes →

normal unhappiness/ reaction to life events
- mood change short term
- have days/times when you feel fine
- still enjoy/look forward to things
- may have difficulty getting off to sleep but, once off, sleep not too badly

Do you really only feel down before periods?
no → yes →

premenstrual tension
- symptoms only/much worse in week or so prior to period
- goes away as soon as period actually starts

Have you been hitting the bottle recently?
no → yes →

alcohol problem
- 'permanent' hangover feeling
- remember alcohol enhances the mood you are in, it doesn't make you happy if you are pissed off

Have you been feeling down for weeks or more?
no → yes →

depression ⚠
- feel down all the time though worse in morning/bit better as day goes on
- no real enjoyment or looking forward to anything
- disturbed sleep or wake early (3–4 a.m. or so) and can't get back to sleep, or increased sleep but wake unrefreshed
- off food/off sex
- if severe, may feel like harming yourself

Do you feel tense and irritable rather than down or depressed?
no → yes →

tension state
- long-term anxiety/stress can make you feel down
- difficulty getting off to sleep or restless/fragmented sleep as likely to wake in night worrying
- on a short fuse

Only rarer causes left, e.g.

drug-related problem from illicit drugs like cannabis, amphetamines

or menopause/premature menopause   **or the Pill**
- lot of flushes/sweats in daytime and hot sweats at night
- periods erratic – missing then flooding/heavy

Remember: ⚠ means see your GP sharpish; ⚠ means an urgent hospital job

Feeling down

'Normal' unhappiness/reaction to life events
Short-term changes in mood are quite normal – some days, for no obvious reason, you're fed up and others you've a spring in your step. Life crises will obviously get you down, but the misery they cause usually sorts itself out given time.

Treatment Time and the support of friends and family are the most helpful 'treatments'. Don't be tempted to turn to drink or drugs – they'll make matters worse. If you're having trouble coping, think about seeing your GP, who might arrange counselling – basically an opportunity to talk through your problems and emotions with someone trained to listen.

Depression
This is a feeling of low mood which lasts for weeks and which you just can't shake off. Other symptoms are usually present (see the chart). Sometimes, it's caused by a nasty life event, though it can start for no obvious reason, and it's very common. Exactly what causes it isn't known, but many doctors now believe it's linked to a lack of a certain chemical in the brain. When severe, it can make people extremely ill, or even suicidal.

Treatment Talk through your problems with family and friends and try the tips described for 'Tension state' below. But if things aren't improving, see your GP. Counselling might help, or she may suggest antidepressants – this treatment really helps, is not addictive, and often has no significant side-effects. It's certainly an improvement on feeling lousy all the time. If you feel suicidal, seek medical help asap – or let those worried about you arrange for you to see the doc if you really can't see the point.

Premenstrual tension
This problem can cause feelings of depression as well as tension. For more details, see the 'Feeling tense' section (p. 64).

Tension state
A constant uptight feeling, usually linked to stress.

Treatment See if you can deal with whatever's winding you up and also try to get on top of the feeling of tension itself. For further details, see the 'Lifestyle/stress' part of the 'Feeling tense' section (p. 64).

Alcohol problem
Overdoing the alcohol can cause depression in two ways – it has a direct chemical effect on the brain and, indirectly, it can create misery through a variety of social catastrophes, such as relationship problems or the loss of your driving licence.

Treatment Cut it down or, better still, out. If you find this difficult, contact your local alcohol unit (try the Yellow Pages or ask at your doctor's surgery) or speak to your GP about the problem.

The Pill
The hormones in the Pill can very occasionally have the side-effect of depression – though this is much less common nowadays as such low doses are used.

Treatment Some women find that vitamin B_6 helps – this is available over the counter, although the available dose is quite low because it has been shown that too much vitamin B_6 can actually be harmful. Otherwise your options are to see if your GP will try you on a different pill or to change your method of family planning completely. Of course, it's tempting and easy to 'blame' the Pill for bouts of depression; in reality, the problem often lies elsewhere, which is worth bearing in mind – not only is it disappointing to find that stopping the Pill makes no difference to your depression, but you have added worry about finding another way of preventing pregnancy!

Drug-related problem
Illicit drug use can cause a low mood. As with alcohol, the effect may be direct (long-term cannabis use can result in apathy, while stopping regular amphetamine use can cause symptoms of depression) or indirect, through a severely disrupted lifestyle.

Treatment Use the same approach as for alcohol – see above.

Menopause/early menopause
Emotional changes, including depression, can be caused or aggravated by the menopause. This is unlikely to be your problem, though, as the menopause usually occurs at an age outside the scope of this book – and if you have an early menopause (especially if this happened under the age of 40), you may well already be on hormone replacement therapy, which should sort out any symptoms the menopause would otherwise have caused.

Treatment If you think the menopause, or an early menopause, is making you feel down, see your GP to discuss the situation.

Feeling tense

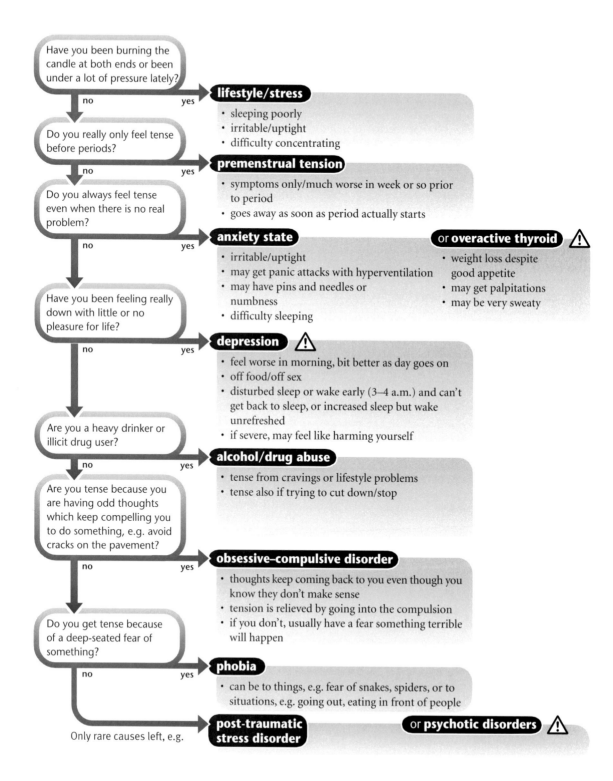

Have you been burning the candle at both ends or been under a lot of pressure lately?

no — yes →

lifestyle/stress

- sleeping poorly
- irritable/uptight
- difficulty concentrating

Do you really only feel tense before periods?

no — yes →

premenstrual tension

- symptoms only/much worse in week or so prior to period
- goes away as soon as period actually starts

Do you always feel tense even when there is no real problem?

no — yes →

anxiety state

- irritable/uptight
- may get panic attacks with hyperventilation
- may have pins and needles or numbness
- difficulty sleeping

or overactive thyroid ⚠

- weight loss despite good appetite
- may get palpitations
- may be very sweaty

Have you been feeling really down with little or no pleasure for life?

no — yes →

depression ⚠

- feel worse in morning, bit better as day goes on
- off food/off sex
- disturbed sleep or wake early (3–4 a.m.) and can't get back to sleep, or increased sleep but wake unrefreshed
- if severe, may feel like harming yourself

Are you a heavy drinker or illicit drug user?

no — yes →

alcohol/drug abuse

- tense from cravings or lifestyle problems
- tense also if trying to cut down/stop

Are you tense because you are having odd thoughts which keep compelling you to do something, e.g. avoid cracks on the pavement?

no — yes →

obsessive–compulsive disorder

- thoughts keep coming back to you even though you know they don't make sense
- tension is relieved by going into the compulsion
- if you don't, usually have a fear something terrible will happen

Do you get tense because of a deep-seated fear of something?

no — yes →

phobia

- can be to things, e.g. fear of snakes, spiders, or to situations, e.g. going out, eating in front of people

Only rare causes left, e.g.

post-traumatic stress disorder

or psychotic disorders ⚠

Feeling tense

Lifestyle/stress Being under pressure – through, for example, relationship, work, or money worries – can make you feel uptight all the time.

Treatment If possible, try to get to the root of the problem by sorting out the stressful areas of your life. Increasing your physical exercise to burn off nervous energy, and cutting down your caffeine intake (e.g. tea, coffee, and cola) may help. Relaxation techniques are worthwhile: basically, this means whatever switches you off. If you're stuck, try a relaxation cassette tape or a self-help book – there are many available. You could also talk to your GP as she might be able to advise you about other relaxation exercises, or send you to see someone to help manage your tension. But don't expect a prescription for a tranquilliser – these are hardly ever used these days.

Premenstrual tension This is a phenomenon which most women will be familiar with to some extent, but although it's a common problem, it's only a minority who are badly affected by it. The feeling of tension building up to – and relieved by – your period may be only one of a number of symptoms you suffer. Others include breast tenderness, bloating, and a worsening of other problems, such as migraine. The precise cause remains a mystery – it's probably a combination of hormonal influences, psychological factors (such as whether you're already feeling down or tense), and social factors (such as how much stress you're under).

Treatment Self-help can get you a long way with this problem. All the measures mentioned above under 'Lifestyle/ stress' are worth trying. If you're getting nowhere and the symptoms are really distressing – or if you think you might be depressed and the premenstrual tension each month is simply the 'last straw' – then discuss the situation with your GP as there are various treatments which might help. It's important not to look for a miracle cure, though – because premenstrual syndrome is caused by a combination of problems, it's unlikely that there will by any 'magic bullet' answer. For advice regarding bloating, or breast pain, see pages 12 and 40, respectively.

Anxiety state A certain level of anxiety in certain circumstances is, of course, normal. But if feelings of anxiety are overwhelming, or continue when they should have settled, or appear for no reason, then they can become a problem. Also, an anxiety state can cause, or show itself through, 'panic attacks' (see the 'Hyperventilation' part of the 'Shortness of breath' section, p. 132).

Treatment The advice given in 'Lifestyle/stress' (above) may help (see also the treatment of panic attacks in the 'Shortness of breath' section, p. 132). If you're not able to get on top of the situation yourself, see your GP. She may be able to help by giving you some advice or by getting you to see someone who will teach you techniques to recognize and control your anxiety (such as a psychologist or a community psychiatric nurse). Tranquillizers are usually avoided if possible, although they may be used for a short while to ease a crisis.

Depression Depression and feeling tense often go hand in hand. For details about depression and its treatment, see the 'Feeling down' section (p. 62).

Alcohol/drug abuse Illicit substances may relax you while you're taking them, but usually end up making you tense – because your body may start to crave them, and because your lifestyle may become chaotic and difficult.

Treatment Cut them down or out. And if you're having problems, contact your GP or the local drug and alcohol unit.

Obsessive–compulsive disorder This is a psychological problem which has three parts. First, an obsession – a thought which keeps coming back to you even though you know it doesn't make sense (e.g. that your hands are covered in germs). Second, a compulsion, which is what the thought makes you do (keep washing your hands). And third, the feeling of tension that the whole thing creates. The cause is unknown.

Treatment If it's becoming a problem, see your GP. She'll either give you some advice or she may send you to see someone who specializes in this type of problem (such as a psychologist). Sometimes, medication is necessary and helpful.

Phobia This is an irrational fear which causes lots of worry. Well-known examples include fear of open spaces (agoraphobia) and fear of spiders (arachnophobia). The cause is often unclear, though it may be linked to some upsetting event in your past.

Treatment If the phobia is a real problem rather than a minor inconvenience, speak to your GP – she may be able to sort you out with some practical advice. Or you may need specialist help from someone skilled at helping people overcome phobias (usually a psychologist).

Post-traumatic stress disorder See the 'Problems sleeping' section (p. 120).

Overactive thyroid See the 'Excess sweating' section (p. 58). A feeling of tension is one of the many symptoms an overactive thyroid can produce.

Psychotic disorders These are illnesses like schizophrenia or mania. They cause a variety of symptoms, including, sometimes, a tension state. For further details, see the 'Odd behaviour' section (p. 108).

Flushing

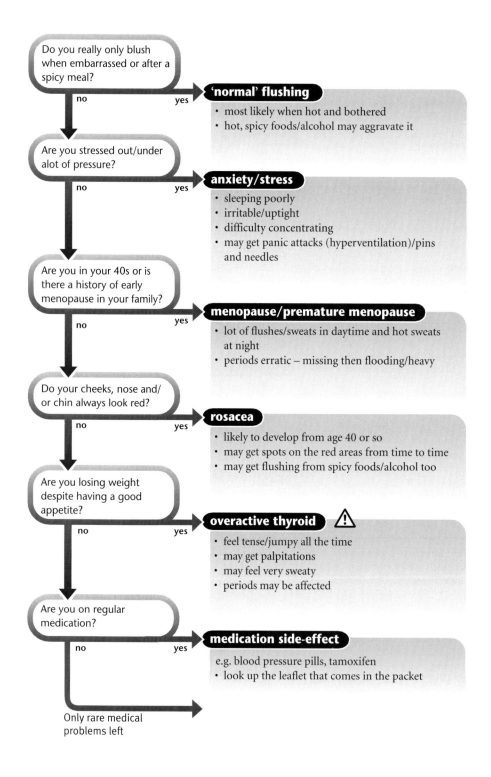

Do you really only blush when embarrassed or after a spicy meal?

no → yes →

'normal' flushing
- most likely when hot and bothered
- hot, spicy foods/alcohol may aggravate it

Are you stressed out/under alot of pressure?

no → yes →

anxiety/stress
- sleeping poorly
- irritable/uptight
- difficulty concentrating
- may get panic attacks (hyperventilation)/pins and needles

Are you in your 40s or is there a history of early menopause in your family?

no → yes →

menopause/premature menopause
- lot of flushes/sweats in daytime and hot sweats at night
- periods erratic – missing then flooding/heavy

Do your cheeks, nose and/or chin always look red?

no → yes →

rosacea
- likely to develop from age 40 or so
- may get spots on the red areas from time to time
- may get flushing from spicy foods/alcohol too

Are you losing weight despite having a good appetite?

no → yes →

overactive thyroid ⚠
- feel tense/jumpy all the time
- may get palpitations
- may feel very sweaty
- periods may be affected

Are you on regular medication?

no → yes →

medication side-effect
e.g. blood pressure pills, tamoxifen
- look up the leaflet that comes in the packet

Only rare medical problems left

'Normal' flushing It's quite normal to blush when embarrassed or feeling self-conscious. Some people tend to blush much more easily than others. This type of flushing is harmless and requires no treatment.

Anxiety and stress If you're uptight you'll tend to blush more easily, or even feel flushed most of the time. You'll probably get other symptoms of tension too, like sweating and palpitations.

Treatment See the 'Feeling tense' section (p. 64).

Menopause/premature menopause At the menopause, or 'change', your ovaries stop producing the hormone oestrogen. This has a number of effects on your body, including flushing, which seems to be caused by the lack of hormones resetting your internal 'thermostat'. Your periods will stop too, although the flushing can start while you're still experiencing a menstrual cycle. The menopause usually happens at around the age of 50. This book is aimed at the 15–45 age group, so if you think your flushes are caused by your ovaries packing up then you may well have a 'premature menopause' (the menopause occurring before the age of 45). This can be brought on by some operations – any surgery in which both your ovaries are removed will definitely cause an early menopause and so, too, may a hysterectomy, even if your ovaries were 'conserved' (not taken away). Some drugs or other treatments for cancer (chemotherapy or radiotherapy) can also permanently stop your ovaries working, but you're unlikely to have had this type of treatment. Often, though, an early menopause happens for no obvious reason.

Treatment Many women experience some flushing at the time of the menopause. The symptom only requires treatment if it's been going on a long time and proving troublesome, in which case you should see your GP. She's likely to discuss with you the pros and cons of hormone replacement therapy (HRT) and will prescribe it if you're keen and it seems appropriate. Lots of symptoms – such as emotional upsets, aches and pains, and tiredness – tend to be put down to the menopause but can be caused by other problems, such as stess and depression. HRT sometimes does give a general feeling of well-being, and should certainly ease flushes caused by the menopause, but shouldn't be seen as a 'cure-all'. There are various aspects of your lifestyle worth considering around the time of the menopause to keep yourself healthy – particularly avoiding smoking, drinking alcohol within sensible limits, taking plenty of exercise, and getting enough calcium in your diet (found particularly in milk, yoghurt, cheese, and sardines).

If you think you're going through an early menopause, you really should see your GP. This is because, quite apart from causing flushes, the lack of oestrogen at a relatively young age can cause problems such as thinning of the bones in later life – this is known as osteoporosis, which can make you more at risk of broken bones when you're older. So in this situation, HRT is a good idea – see your GP so she can check whether or not you really are going through an early menopause and to discuss treatment. If you do start HRT, you're likely to stay on it at least until you reach the usual age of the menopause (around 50). Don't forget to sort out the lifestyle measures mentioned above, too.

It's also important to continue with contraception for a while, unless, of course, you or your partner have been sterilized: contraception is needed for two years after your last period if they stop before the age of 50 and for one year if they stop beyond that age. HRT does not act as a contraceptive.

Rosacea Flushing is one of the symptoms of this skin problem. For further details and advice on treatment, see the 'Rash on the face' section (p. 128).

Overactive thyroid This illness causes a number of symptoms, including flushing. For further details, see the 'Excess sweating' section (p. 58).

Medication side-effect Some prescribed medications – particularly some blood pressure pills and the anti-breast cancer drug tamoxifen – can cause flushing.

Treatment If the flushing is a real nuisance and you think your medication might be the cause, discuss the situation with your GP as she may be able to alter your treatment.

Medical rarities Various rare medical conditions can cause flushing, although there are usually various other symptoms too.

Treatment It's very unlikely that you'd have one of these rare problems. If you're concerned, speak to your GP – she'll arrange any necessary tests.

Hair loss

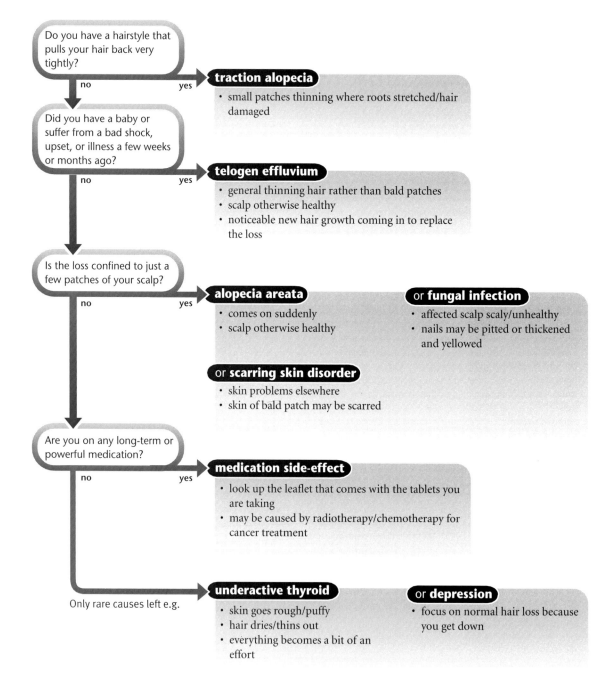

Do you have a hairstyle that pulls your hair back very tightly?

no → yes →

traction alopecia
- small patches thinning where roots stretched/hair damaged

Did you have a baby or suffer from a bad shock, upset, or illness a few weeks or months ago?

no → yes →

telogen effluvium
- general thinning hair rather than bald patches
- scalp otherwise healthy
- noticeable new hair growth coming in to replace the loss

Is the loss confined to just a few patches of your scalp?

no → yes →

alopecia areata
- comes on suddenly
- scalp otherwise healthy

or **fungal infection**
- affected scalp scaly/unhealthy
- nails may be pitted or thickened and yellowed

or **scarring skin disorder**
- skin problems elsewhere
- skin of bald patch may be scarred

Are you on any long-term or powerful medication?

no → yes →

medication side-effect
- look up the leaflet that comes with the tablets you are taking
- may be caused by radiotherapy/chemotherapy for cancer treatment

Only rare causes left e.g.

underactive thyroid
- skin goes rough/puffy
- hair dries/thins out
- everything becomes a bit of an effort

or **depression**
- focus on normal hair loss because you get down

Traction alopecia Some hairstyles, in which hair is pulled back tightly, exert too much pull ('traction') on the hair. As a result, the stretched hair becomes thin and eventually breaks. As this process is repeated, small patches of baldness can develop ('traction alopecia').

Treatment This simply involves altering the offending hairstyle.

Telogen effluvium A human form of moulting. It is usually caused by some 'event' occurring about three months previously: this may be a lifestyle change such as a crash diet, a 'trauma' such as childbirth, or some other illness or psychological upset. As there is a delay of some months before the event leads to hair loss, a connection between the two often isn't made.

Treatment Don't waste your money or time on anything – your hair will be back to normal after about three months of moulting.

Alopecia areata Bald patches with a normal-looking scalp. The cause is unknown and it sometimes runs in families. Occasionally, it results in complete baldness – even, in extreme cases, loss of all body hair and problems with the nails too.

Treatment The good news is that the problem usually sorts itself out in time, usually over a year or so. The bad news is that, if it doesn't, treatment doesn't usually help much. You may be referred to a dermatologist, but more in hope than expectation: although treatments such as creams and injections into the scalp are often tried, their effects are usually very disappointing. Certain patterns of alopecia tend to last longest or get worse. These include people with several patches, loss of eyebrows and eyelashes, previous attacks, and loss of hair at the back of the head.

Medication side-effect Some treatments can cause hair loss. Most people know that powerful drugs given for cancer (chemotherapy) often result in baldness: you're highly unlikely to face this particular problem. Other drugs, such as blood thinning or anti-thyroid medications, can have the same effect.

Treatment If you think that a treatment you're taking is causing hair loss, discuss the situation with whoever is prescribing it – your GP or specialist.

Fungal infection Fungi – microscopic moulds – can get into the scalp and affect the hair. Commonly known as 'ringworm', the infection causes scaling with patches of baldness. It is much more common in children than adults.

Treatment See your GP for a course of anti-fungal pills.

Rare disorders A variety of medical problems, such as anaemia and an underactive thyroid, can cause hair loss. The chances that these will come to light through baldness, though, is remote.

Treatment If your doctor suspects a medical problem, she'll arrange the necessary blood tests and will treat you according to the results.

Scarring skin disorders Any skin diseases which cause scarring can lead to patches of hair loss because hair won't grow where there are scars. These diseases are all very rare.

Treatment You're sure to be referred to a skin specialist for treatment.

Depression If you're feeling down, you may focus on minor annoyances which otherwise wouldn't bother you – such as the small amounts of hair lost when brushing each day. Because you're at a low ebb, you end up blowing this hair loss out of all proportion, becoming convinced that you're losing abnormally large amounts or about to become bald.

Treatment The key thing here is to shift the emphasis from the apparent hair loss to the real problem – the depression. This may be difficult for you to do, but if family or friends repeatedly tell you that you're focusing on the wrong thing and need help with your depression, it's worth letting them persuade you to discuss the situation with your GP. Further advice can be found in the 'Feeling down' section (p. 62).

Headache

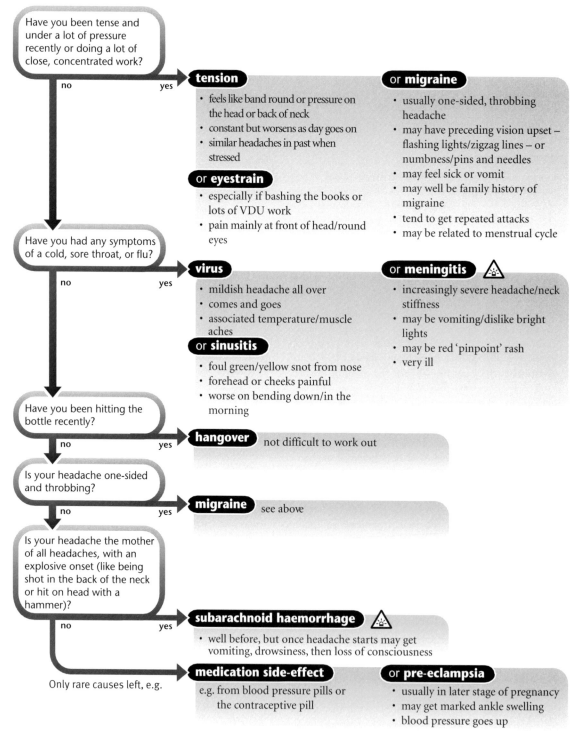

⚠ If you get a sudden severe headache/pain in the back of your neck, or increasing headache and neck stiffness, seek medical help immediately to check for subarachnoid haemorrhage or meningitis.

⚠ If you are on the Pill, or pregnant, and develop a new kind of headache or what seems to be a first migraine attack, then seek medical help ASAP.

Virus A germ, causing a cold or flu. Headache is just part of the all-round grotty feeling that these germs cause.

Treatment Regular paracetamol or aspirin and plenty of fluids.

Tension headache Stress makes the muscles tense, especially on the forehead and in the neck. The tense muscles become tender, causing headache.

Treatment Massage, relaxation, and physical exercise will all help – see also the 'Feeling tense' section (p. 64). Avoid painkillers if possible as they can actually make it worse.

Migraine Migraine is caused by the blood vessels to the brain opening wide – blood pumps through, causing a pounding headache. The cause is unknown, but it often runs in families, and attacks can be linked to diet, stress, or tiredness, and the Pill.

Treatment An attack of migraine needs rest and quiet, and strongish painkillers such as paracetamol and codeine combinations (available from the chemist without prescription). Soluble ones are often the most effective and quickest to work – it's always important to take painkillers as soon as you feel your migraine coming on. If you get repeated attacks, try to figure out – and avoid – whatever brings them on. It's usually pretty obvious if it's something in your diet (such as cheese, chocolate, or red wine). Missing meals can also provoke attacks, so try to eat regularly. It's worth seeing your GP if the painkillers described above don't help or if you're getting very frequent attacks (say more than one a fortnight) – in both cases, she'll be able to prescribe treatment to help. If you're on the Pill, the following situations should make you stop it and discuss matters further with your GP: your first-ever severe migraine, a migraine which goes on getting worse and worse, or migraine with 'neurological' effects (which means numbness or weakness down one side of your face or body, speech disturbance, or loss of part of your vision). If your migraine only happens in your week off the Pill, it's worth trying the 'tricycle' regime – see below under 'Medication side-effect'.

Sinusitis This is an infection of the sinuses, which are air spaces in your forehead and cheeks. The infection causes a build-up of pressure, resulting in pain over the affected sinus. If you tend to suffer a blocked nose most of the time, you might keep getting attacks of sinusitis.

Treatment Painkillers and steam inhalations, and see your GP if there's no improvement within a few days, as you may need antibiotics. You might also need some treatment to clear your nose if you keep getting attacks – being stuffed up all the time tends to block the sinuses, leading to repeated infections. This can be treated with either nose sprays or surgery.

Eyestrain If you can't see clearly, you'll tend to keep screwing your eyes up. This makes the muscles around the eyes sore, causing headache.

Treatment See an optician.

Hangover Figuring out why you've got a stonking headache – along with various other symptoms – the morning after the night before isn't exactly rocket science.

Treatment Dose yourself up with fluids (preferably fruit juice) and painkillers, and maybe some antacid if your stomach feels 'acidic'. Preventive measures in the future include avoiding binges and drinking plenty of water before crashing out.

(**Medication side-effect**) Some prescribed treatments, such as blood pressure pills, can cause headaches. Ironically, so can painkillers (even those bought over the counter) if used regularly. The Pill can also occasionally cause headache as a side-effect.

Treatment Speak to your GP if you think a prescribed treatment is giving you headaches. And go easy on the painkillers. If you've only recently started the Pill, it's worth persevering as the problem may settle (but see the warnings about migraine, above). Some women only get headaches in the week off the Pill (the 'pill-free week'). In this case, you can try what doctors call the 'tricycle' regime, which means taking four packs continuously (with no pill-free week) and only then having a seven-day break; you then repeat the process with four continuous packs and so on. This method is safe and reliable and means you only have four 'periods' a year, so you suffer four rather than 12 headaches. The only other alternative, if the headaches are really bothering you, is to change your Pill or your family planning method.

(**Subarachnoid haemorrhage**) A burst blood vessel in the brain. Very serious and very rare.

Treatment Go straight to hospital.

(**Meningitis**) An infection of the lining of the brain. Also serious, but rarer than you'd think, considering the media coverage it gets.

Treatment This needs immediate attention. Call your doctor or go to hospital – whichever is likely to be quickest.

(**Other rare medical problems**) Some small-print problems, including an unusual type of migraine called 'cluster headache', brain tumours, and extremely high blood pressure (especially during pregnancy, when it is called 'pre-eclampsia'), can cause headaches.

Treatment Problems like these are thankfully very rare, though the average patient is often worried about them by the times she decides to see her GP. So if you do visit the doc, anticipate lots of reassurance rather than a brain scan.

Heavy periods

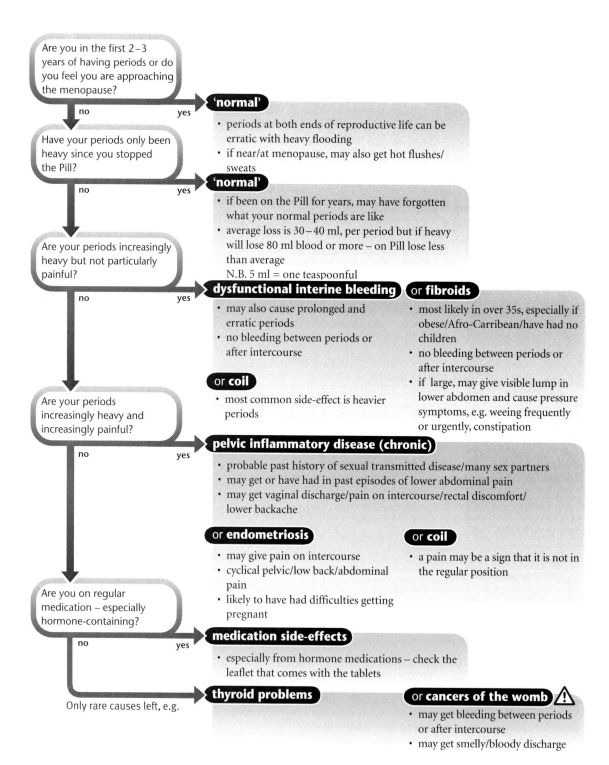

Are you in the first 2–3 years of having periods or do you feel you are approaching the menopause?

no → [down]   yes →

'normal'
- periods at both ends of reproductive life can be erratic with heavy flooding
- if near/at menopause, may also get hot flushes/sweats

Have your periods only been heavy since you stopped the Pill?

no → [down]   yes →

'normal'
- if been on the Pill for years, may have forgotten what your normal periods are like
- average loss is 30–40 ml, per period but if heavy will lose 80 ml blood or more – on Pill lose less than average
  N.B. 5 ml = one teaspoonful

Are your periods increasingly heavy but not particularly painful?

no → [down]   yes →

dysfunctional interine bleeding
- may also cause prolonged and erratic periods
- no bleeding between periods or after intercourse

or fibroids
- most likely in over 35s, especially if obese/Afro-Carribean/have had no children
- no bleeding between periods or after intercourse
- if large, may give visible lump in lower abdomen and cause pressure symptoms, e.g. weeing frequently or urgently, constipation

or coil
- most common side-effect is heavier periods

Are your periods increasingly heavy and increasingly painful?

no → [down]   yes →

pelvic inflammatory disease (chronic)
- probable past history of sexual transmitted disease/many sex partners
- may get or have had in past episodes of lower abdominal pain
- may get vaginal discharge/pain on intercourse/rectal discomfort/lower backache

or endometriosis
- may give pain on intercourse
- cyclical pelvic/low back/abdominal pain
- likely to have had difficulties getting pregnant

or coil
- a pain may be a sign that it is not in the regular position

Are you on regular medication – especially hormone-containing?

no → [down]   yes →

medication side-effects
- especially from hormone medications – check the leaflet that comes with the tablets

Only rare causes left, e.g.

thyroid problems

or cancers of the womb ⚠
- may get bleeding between periods or after intercourse
- may get smelly/bloody discharge

'Normal' How heavy you feel your periods are depends on how much blood is actually lost and what you believe you should reasonably expect or tolerate: what one woman might regard as perfectly OK, another may view as completely unacceptable. Research in hospital has shown that only 40% of women seeing specialists because of heavy periods actually suffer what is medically defined as 'excessive' bleeding. Periods do tend to be heavier around the ages of puberty and the menopause and will appear to be heavier if you have come off the Pill, as this usually makes periods lighter.

Treatment If you believe your periods are heavy, an over-the-counter treatment such as ibuprofen may help (it helps period pains too). If this doesn't work, and you really do feel your periods are intolerable, it's worth seeing your GP. She can examine you to ensure there's no serious problem, and can try to make some assessment of whether your periods are really abnormally heavy – for example, by taking a blood test to see if the bleeding has made you anaemic. If you need contraception as well, then going on the Pill should sort all your problems out.

Dysfunctional uterine bleeding In about half of cases of genuinely heavy periods, no particular cause is found. This type of bleeding is known as 'dysfunctional'.

Treatment Ibuprofen (available from the chemist) can cut down the bleeding – take it as early as possible, then regularly until the period stops. If it doesn't help then see your GP, who will check you over to confirm the diagnosis and to discuss other treatments – such as other anti-inflammatory drugs, pills to help the blood clot, hormone treatments (such as the Pill – particularly if you also need to sort out your family planning), or a type of hormone-releasing coil (see below). If these treatments don't work, the problem is severe, and you might consider surgery, your GP may refer you to a gynaecologist.

Fibroids These are benign growths of the muscle layer of the womb. They are very common and eventually shrink after the menopause.

Treatment Your GP may try some of the tablet treatments described for dysfunctional bleeding (see above). But if these don't work, your fibroids are very large, and you have a long wait before you get to the menopause, you'll probably need to see a gynaecologist for possible surgery.

Intrauterine contraceptive device ('the coil') The coil usually consists of a small piece of plastic encased in some copper. It is inserted through the cervix (neck of the womb) into the womb and needs replacing every four years or so. It is a very effective contraceptive but it may make the periods heavier (and more painful).

Treatment If you've only had your coil for a few months and are otherwise happy with it, it's worth waiting and seeing – this problem often settles on its own. Some of the tablet treatments used for dysfunctional uterine bleeding (see above) can help persistent heavy bleeding, particularly if you're keen to hang on to your coil. But if all else fails, the only solution is to have this particular coil removed and sort out another form of contraception – there now exists a new type of hormone-releasing coil which makes periods lighter (or even stops them altogether), so this might be an option.

Chronic pelvic inflammatory disease This is explained, and the treatment discussed, in the 'Lower abdominal pain – recurrent' section (p. 94). Some of the treatments mentioned above for dysfunctional uterine bleeding may help the heavy periods.

Endometriosis This is explained, and the treatment discussed, in the 'Lower abdominal pain – recurrent' section (p. 94).

Medication side-effect Some prescribed medications can cause heavy periods as a side-effect. These include blood thinning pills (which you're unlikely to be on), the Pill (which you may well be taking but which, if anything, usually lightens the periods), and hormone replacement therapy (which you're also unlikely to be taking, unless you've had an early menopause).

Treatment If you think your medication might be causing your heavy periods, see your GP. She might be able to stop your treatment or provide you with an alternative.

Other rare problems Thyroid problems, disorders of blood clotting, and polyps or cancers of the lining of the womb can all very rarely cause heavy periods.

Treatment You are very unlikely to have any of these illnesses – but if you're concerned, see your GP, who will arrange any necessary tests.

High temperature

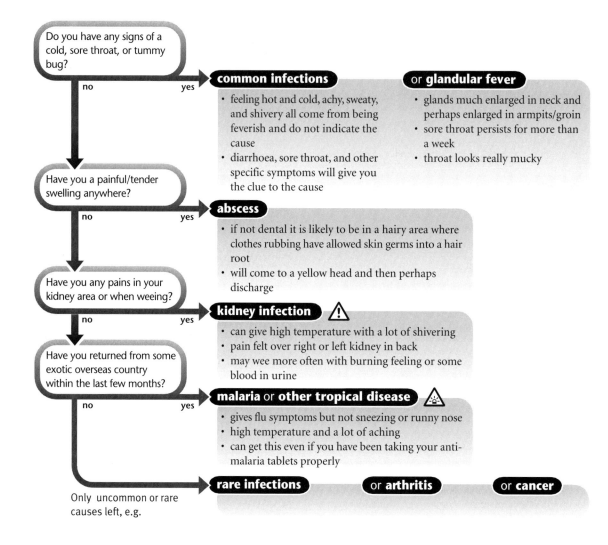

Do you have any signs of a cold, sore throat, or tummy bug?

no — yes

common infections
- feeling hot and cold, achy, sweaty, and shivery all come from being feverish and do not indicate the cause
- diarrhoea, sore throat, and other specific symptoms will give you the clue to the cause

or glandular fever
- glands much enlarged in neck and perhaps enlarged in armpits/groin
- sore throat persists for more than a week
- throat looks really mucky

Have you a painful/tender swelling anywhere?

no — yes

abscess
- if not dental it is likely to be in a hairy area where clothes rubbing have allowed skin germs into a hair root
- will come to a yellow head and then perhaps discharge

Have you any pains in your kidney area or when weeing?

no — yes

kidney infection ⚠
- can give high temperature with a lot of shivering
- pain felt over right or left kidney in back
- may wee more often with burning feeling or some blood in urine

Have you returned from some exotic overseas country within the last few months?

no — yes

malaria or **other tropical disease** ⚠
- gives flu symptoms but not sneezing or runny nose
- high temperature and a lot of aching
- can get this even if you have been taking your anti-malaria tablets properly

rare infections   or **arthritis**   or **cancer**

Only uncommon or rare causes left, e.g.

⚠ If you have a high temperature and feel more and more ill with increasing headache/neck stiffness/vomiting, or if you develop a red pinpoint rash, then seek medical help immediately to check for meningitis.

Remember: ⚠ means see your GP sharpish; ⚠ means an urgent hospital job

Common infections These include colds, tonsillitis, chest infections, flu, and tummy bugs, which can all cause a high temperature for a few days. Pushing your temperature up is actually one of the ways your body tries to fight off these germs – the fever fries the bug and also makes your immune defences work faster.

Treatment The temperature itself needs no treatment at all, though you'll feel more comfortable if you keep yourself as cool as possible and take regular paracetamol and plenty of fluids. Otherwise, it's a question of sorting out the infection which is causing the high temperature. Most (including colds, the flu, and most tummy bugs) are caused by viruses, which usually settle on their own in a few days – there's no magic cure for these infections. Some, such as tonsillitis and chest infections, may be helped by antibiotics – see the 'Sore throat', (p. 136) and 'Cough' (p. 46) sections.

Glandular fever This is explained, and its treatment outlined, in the 'Sore throat' section (p. 136).

Abscess Abscesses are infections which develop into lumps of pus, like very large and painful boils. They can appear anywhere on the body, especially in hairy areas and around the back passage. They can also develop inside the body – this is much more unusual but can happen, for example, after a severe chest or kidney infection. Your temperature will tend to go up and down until the abscess clears up.

Treatment An early abscess may be cured by antibiotics. Otherwise, it'll need lancing – see your GP or go to casualty. Internal abscesses are obviously more complicated and need hospital treatment, which your GP will arrange.

Kidney infection A germ getting into your kidney will push your temperature up and cause other symptoms too. This is pretty unusual and can be a sign of some other problem with your waterworks, such as kidney stones.

Treatment You need to see your GP asap for treatment with antibiotics. Drinking plenty of fluids will help too. If you're really rough with it, and vomiting, you may need to go to hospital. You may also need further tests once you're better to work out why you developed a kidney infection in the first place.

Malaria (and other tropical diseases) People very occasionally bring back exotic illnesses as unpleasant souvenirs of their travels abroad. A few of these – and some types of malaria in particular – develop slowly and may cause a high temperature which keeps coming back, before any other symptoms develop.

Treatment If you've been somewhere exotic and you've developed a persistent fever which has no obvious cause (like a cold or sore throat), see your GP asap, especially if you feel really rough too. Do this even if you've taken anti-malaria pills or it's been some months since you travelled: malaria can take quite a while to develop, and the pills taken to prevent it aren't 100% effective. Besides, you may have some exotic infection other than malaria. If your GP thinks you may have brought home an unusual germ of this sort, she'll either arrange some urgent blood tests or send you to hospital.

Cancer Any cancer can cause a recurring high temperature. An example is lymphoma (see the 'Swollen glands' section, p. 142). Most other cancers produce other symptoms which give the game away.

Treatment It's most unlikely that your temperature is caused by anything nasty – but if you're worried, see your GP.

Rare infections Some serious and unusual infections, such as meningitis and septicaemia (blood poisoning), can cause a sudden high temperature as your body tries to fight them off. There are likely to be other symptoms too, and you'll be feeling seriously ill. Some other rare but important infections don't come on so dramatically. Examples include TB and infection with the HIV virus (the cause of AIDS). These types of germs can cause a prolonged or recurrent fever and usually make you feel gradually more unwell.

Treatment Meningitis and blood poisoning require immediate treatment in hospital. If you're worried you might have TB or HIV infection, you need to see your GP soon to discuss the situation – she will arrange any necessary tests.

Arthritis Rheumatoid arthritis and some other rare types of arthritis – but not the common 'wear and tear' sort (osteoarthritis) – can give you a recurrent high temperature, amongst other symptoms.

Treatment See your GP. She will refer you to a joint specialist (a rheumatologist). For further information, see the 'Rheumatoid arthritis' part of the 'Multiple joint pains' section (p. 100).

Other uncommon medical conditions Problems that can very occasionally cause a prolonged temperature include inflammatory bowel disease (see the 'Diarrhoea' section, p. 50) and the side-effects of medication.

Treatment Talk to your GP if you think you might have one of these rare causes.

Hoarse voice

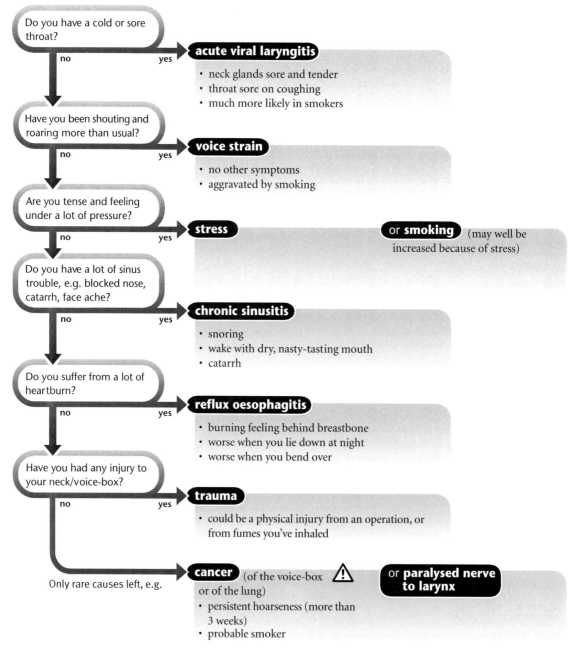

Do you have a cold or sore throat?
no / **yes**

acute viral laryngitis
- neck glands sore and tender
- throat sore on coughing
- much more likely in smokers

Have you been shouting and roaring more than usual?
no / **yes**

voice strain
- no other symptoms
- aggravated by smoking

Are you tense and feeling under a lot of pressure?
no / **yes**

stress   **or smoking** (may well be increased because of stress)

Do you have a lot of sinus trouble, e.g. blocked nose, catarrh, face ache?
no / **yes**

chronic sinusitis
- snoring
- wake with dry, nasty-tasting mouth
- catarrh

Do you suffer from a lot of heartburn?
no / **yes**

reflux oesophagitis
- burning feeling behind breastbone
- worse when you lie down at night
- worse when you bend over

Have you had any injury to your neck/voice-box?
no / **yes**

trauma
- could be a physical injury from an operation, or from fumes you've inhaled

Only rare causes left, e.g.

cancer (of the voice-box ⚠ or of the lung)   **or paralysed nerve to larynx**
- persistent hoarseness (more than 3 weeks)
- probable smoker

⚠ If you have persistent hoarseness lasting more than 3 weeks, see your GP so she can rule out cancer of the voice-box.

Remember: ⚠ means see your GP sharpish; ⚠ means an urgent hospital job

Acute viral laryngitis The common germs which cause colds and sore throats can inflame the voice-box (or larynx), causing hoarseness.

Treatment Try some simple self-help measures like hot drinks, steam inhalations, and paracetamol while you're waiting the few days for the problem to settle. Also, avoid cigarette smoke and go easy on your voice – so no shouting or lengthy phone conversations. Antibiotics don't usually help this problem, but if you also get a bad cough with a lot of green or yellow spit, you may be developing a chest infection (see 'Cough' section, p. 46) which might be helped by a short course.

Voice strain There are two types. The 'acute' sort simply means you've strained your voice-box by screaming or shouting. You don't need a doctor to tell you that shouting to make yourself heard at a party can leave you hoarse for a day or two. The 'chronic' sort is caused by continuous voice strain – such as untrained singing – and makes the voice hoarse, to some extent, most of the time. Sometimes, this can result in small lumps ('singer's nodules') on the vocal cords.

Treatment Chronic voice strain will only be cured if you either stop whatever is upsetting your voice-box, or start doing it properly. So if you're a singer with this problem, try getting some voice training. If the hoarseness has been there for ages, and continues despite your best efforts, you might have singer's nodules. Ear, Nose, and Throat ('ENT') surgeons can deal with these quite easily, so discuss the situation with your GP.

Smoking Cigarette smoke irritates the vocal cords, making them swell slightly. This can make the voice constantly hoarse.

Treatment Stopping smoking should sort the problem out, unless you're also abusing your vocal cords in some other way (see 'Voice strain', above). But it's important to get persistent and otherwise unexplained hoarseness checked out further, especially if you're a smoker – so speak to your GP.

Stress Small muscles in the voice-box help produce the sounds of your voice. If you're uptight, these muscles get tense and so don't produce the sounds properly. This usually happens in certain stressful situations, like making a speech or giving a presentation; sometimes, if you're very tense all the time, the voice tends to stay hoarse.

Treatment Try the relaxation advice given in the 'Anxiety' part of the 'Palpitations' section (p. 116). Voice training may help if your voice only lets you down in certain stressful situations.

Chronic sinusitis The sinuses are air spaces in the skull. If you have some problem with your nose – such as a blockage caused by polyps, allergy, or an old injury – the drainage system of the sinuses may not work properly. This causes the sinuses to fill with fluid, which gets infected and tends to drip down the back of the throat, causing catarrh and an inflamed voice-box.

Treatment Self-help measures include steam inhalations and stopping smoking. If your nose is blocked or runs a lot of the time, you could try an anti-allergy nose spray from the chemist such as beclomethasone. If you're getting nowhere and the symptom is a real nuisance, see your GP – she may try some other treatments or she may refer you to an ENT surgeon for possible surgery to unblock your nose.

Trauma Any damage to the voice-box will cause hoarseness. Possibilities include a punch, accidentally breathing in hot steam or chemical fumes, and any operation under anaesthetic (because of the large tube put down your throat during surgery).

Treatment The hoarseness will right itself after a few days. Seek medical attention urgently if a blow to the throat, or inhaling something nasty, is making it hard to breathe.

Damaged nerve to larynx If this nerve is damaged, then one or both of your vocal cords will be paralysed. This has a number of very rare causes.

Treatment Your GP is certain to send you to an ENT specialist to get the problem sorted out.

Reflux oesophagitis This is explained in the 'Indigestion' section (p. 78). It can result in hoarseness if the acid comes right up the gullet into the voice-box, where it causes an irritation.

Treatment See the 'Indigestion' section (p. 78).

Cancer Highly unlikely in the under 50s, and incredibly unlikely in non-smokers.

Treatment See your GP, who will send you for an urgent appointment at the hospital if she's concerned.

Indigestion

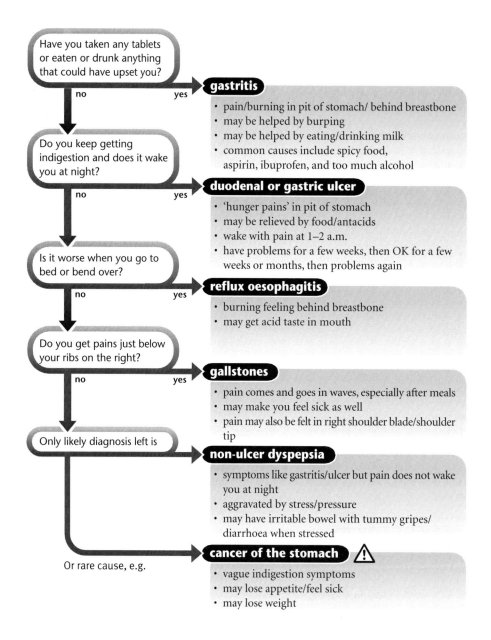

Have you taken any tablets or eaten or drunk anything that could have upset you?

gastritis
- pain/burning in pit of stomach/ behind breastbone
- may be helped by burping
- may be helped by eating/drinking milk
- common causes include spicy food, aspirin, ibuprofen, and too much alcohol

Do you keep getting indigestion and does it wake you at night?

duodenal or gastric ulcer
- 'hunger pains' in pit of stomach
- may be relieved by food/antacids
- wake with pain at 1–2 a.m.
- have problems for a few weeks, then OK for a few weeks or months, then problems again

Is it worse when you go to bed or bend over?

reflux oesophagitis
- burning feeling behind breastbone
- may get acid taste in mouth

Do you get pains just below your ribs on the right?

gallstones
- pain comes and goes in waves, especially after meals
- may make you feel sick as well
- pain may also be felt in right shoulder blade/shoulder tip

Only likely diagnosis left is

non-ulcer dyspepsia
- symptoms like gastritis/ulcer but pain does not wake you at night
- aggravated by stress/pressure
- may have irritable bowel with tummy gripes/diarrhoea when stressed

Or rare cause, e.g.

cancer of the stomach ⚠
- vague indigestion symptoms
- may lose appetite/feel sick
- may lose weight

Gastritis The stomach produces acid to help digest the food. But sometimes the acid can inflame the stomach lining ('gastritis'), causing indigestion. There are a number of things which can stir up acid problems. The commonest is alcohol – this is why indigestion is a familiar part of a hangover. Some tablets, such as aspirin and anti-inflammatory drugs (like ibuprofen), can have the same effect.

Treatment If this is a one-off problem – such as after an alcohol binge – just drink plenty of water and take some antacids from the chemist. But if you keep getting problems, look at your diet and lifestyle. Avoid spicy foods, eat regularly, and cut down cigarettes and alcohol. Also, steer clear of acidic over-the-counter painkillers like aspirin and ibuprofen; paracetamol is OK. Antacids – used when needed – are usually very helpful.

Duodenal or gastric ulcer Occasionally, the acid burns a small crater in the lining of the tube which carries food away from the stomach (a duodenal ulcer) or, less commonly, in the stomach itself (a gastric ulcer). This type of problem sometimes runs in families and may be brought on, or aggravated by, the things discussed above.

Treatment This is explained in the 'Gastritis/ulcer' part of the 'Abdominal pain – recurrent' section (p. 10).

Non-ulcer dyspepsia This gives all the symptoms of acidity or ulcers but is caused by something else – probably the muscles of the stomach and gullet squeezing too hard or in an uncoordinated way. So it's a bit like 'irritable bowel syndrome' (see the 'Abdominal pain – recurrent' section, p. 10). In fact, many people with non-ulcer dyspepsia also get irritable bowel syndrome, and some doctors think they're actually the same thing. The cause is unknown, but it may be linked to stress.

Treatment It's sensible to look at the lifestyle areas discussed above. Antacids do seem to help some people, even though it's not really caused by excess acid. If your symp-
toms do seem to be stress related, try to sort out whatever is winding you up and do some relaxation therapy (see the 'Feeling tense' section, p. 64). It's worth seeing your GP if you're getting nowhere: she might try more powerful acid-suppressant pills or medication to relax the muscles in your stomach and gullet. There may be no 'magic bullet', though, so you may have to accept that you'll get some symptoms from time to time.

Reflux oesophagitis Acid sits in the stomach, waiting to digest food, and is prevented from entering the gullet by a valve. If this valve doesn't work perfectly, the acid can rise into the gullet, inflaming its lining ('reflux oesophagitis'). This is usually felt as a burning in the centre of the chest ('heartburn'), which can lead to indigestion.

Treatment You can make a variety of tweaks to your lifestyle which should help. These include: shedding some pounds if you're overweight; taking care not to overdo the spicy foods and alcohol; cutting down, or stopping, smoking; not eating too late in the evening; raising the head of your bed by a few inches; and avoiding acidic over-the-counter painkillers like aspirin and ibuprofen. Antacid mixtures from the chemist can help if you get a lot of heartburn; if they don't work, more powerful treatments are available from your GP.

Gallstones These are discussed, and their treatment explained, in the 'Abdominal pain – one-off' section (p. 8). They can cause an indigestion-type pain, especially after fatty meals.

Stomach cancer Relax. This is rare in the under 50s.

Treatment It's extremely unlikely that you've got this problem unless you're over 50. Speak to your GP if you're concerned. If she's in any doubt, she'll arrange for a specialist at the hospital to take a look into your stomach with a narrow, flexible telescope (called an 'endoscope').

Infertility

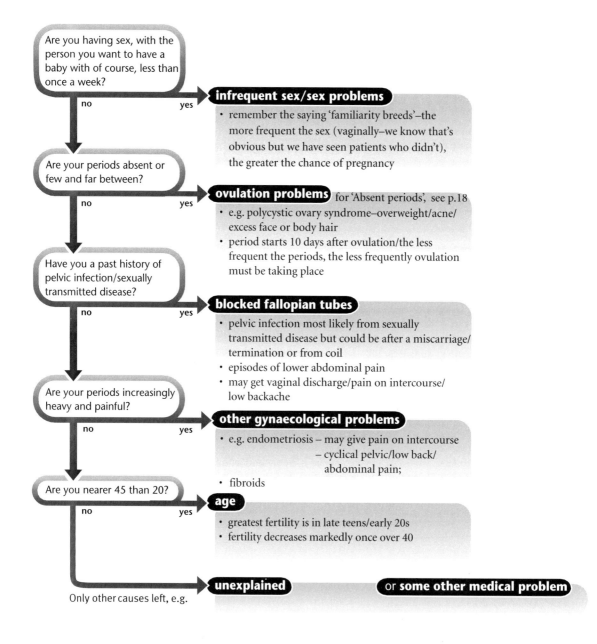

Are you having sex, with the person you want to have a baby with of course, less than once a week?

no → yes

infrequent sex/sex problems
- remember the saying 'familiarity breeds'–the more frequent the sex (vaginally–we know that's obvious but we have seen patients who didn't), the greater the chance of pregnancy

Are your periods absent or few and far between?

no → yes

ovulation problems for 'Absent periods', see p.18
- e.g. polycystic ovary syndrome–overweight/acne/ excess face or body hair
- period starts 10 days after ovulation/the less frequent the periods, the less frequently ovulation must be taking place

Have you a past history of pelvic infection/sexually transmitted disease?

no → yes

blocked fallopian tubes
- pelvic infection most likely from sexually transmitted disease but could be after a miscarriage/ termination or from coil
- episodes of lower abdominal pain
- may get vaginal discharge/pain on intercourse/ low backache

Are your periods increasingly heavy and painful?

no → yes

other gynaecological problems
- e.g. endometriosis – may give pain on intercourse – cyclical pelvic/low back/ abdominal pain;
- fibroids

Are you nearer 45 than 20?

no → yes

age
- greatest fertility is in late teens/early 20s
- fertility decreases markedly once over 40

unexplained   **or some other medical problem**

Only other causes left, e.g.

NB 1. Most couples will manage to achieve a pregnancy within a year of trying – and those who don't usually succeed in the second year. Often, the cause is a combination of problems in both the man and the woman, rather than the cause lying with one or the other – so it's best to view it as a joint problem and, if you decide to see your GP, to go together. She'll assess the situation and is likley to arrange a sperm test for your partner while she checks you out too.

2. If you've been trying without success for a couple of years or so, and you're really keen on falling pregnant, your GP is likely to refer you for specialist help regardless of the specific cause of the problem. And you may get referred earlier than this if you're over 35 or seem to have some gynaecological problem which might be causing the infertility.

3. While you're thinking about sorting out your infertility, don't forget some basic lifestyle measures: for example, cut down on the alcohol and avoid cigarettes. Start eating plenty of the vitamin 'folic acid' (found in brown bread, bananas, broccoli, and bran flakes, among other things) and start taking a supplement of the same vitamin (folic acid, 400 microgram strength, once a day – available from the chemist), as this helps protect against spina bifida when you do fall pregnant. Also, check that you have been immunized against German measles – if not, arrange for this to be done via your GP (although you must not fall pregnant within three months of having the immunization, so you'll need to use contraception to cover this period).

Infrequent sex/sexual problems
Pressure of work, night shifts, or simply feeling exhausted may mean that one or both of you haven't the time or energy for sex. Or you may have some other problem affecting your love life, such as a general loss of sex drive. Obviously, the less often you have sex, the less likely you are to fall pregnant.

Treatment Couples seriously wanting to start a family should aim to have sex at least two or three times a week, which will probably be music to his ears. But slavishly sticking to set rules like this, or timing when you should have sex using fertility kits, can cause more problems than they solve by messing up the spontaneity of your love life and causing stress. For more information about a loss of interest in sex, see the 'Loss of sex drive' section (p. 90).

Ovulation problems
If your ovaries don't release an egg each month then, obviously, you're unlikely to fall pregnant. There are a number of reasons why this might happen. Most make the periods pack up or become very scanty, and are explained in the 'Absent periods' section (p. 18).

Treatment You need to see your GP. She is likely to run some tests to see why you aren't having any periods and, if nothing obvious shows up that she can sort out, will refer you to a gynaecologist for specialized treatment to help you ovulate.

Blocked fallopian tubes
An egg is released, each month, by your ovaries and travels down the 'fallopian tube' en route to your womb. If this tube is blocked then it won't be able to meet up with incoming sperm, so you'll have problems falling pregnant. The block may be caused by previous infections or surgery, or by some other problem.

Treatment Again, you'll already be under specialist care by the time your doctor works out that this is the problem. Surgery to unblock the tube may be offered, but the results are not very good. It's more likely that you'll be offered the specialized types of 'assisted conception' used in the various other forms of infertility.

Some other gynaecological problems
Fibroids, endometriosis, and some other gynaecological problems can affect fertility. Endometriosis is explained further in the 'Painful periods' section (p. 114); fibroids are discussed fully in the 'Heavy periods' section (p. 72).

Treatment Sometimes, treatment 'aimed' directly at the problem (such as surgery for fibroids or hormone treatment for endometriosis) may solve the infertility. More commonly, the focus is on the infertility itself, and specialized techniques will be used by your gynaecologist to help you fall pregnant.

Unexplained
Despite thorough testing of both partners, the cause of infertility can remain unclear.

Treatment If you fall into this category then you're likely already to be under the care of a gynaecologist, who will do his or her best to help you fall pregnant with specialist treatment.

Age
Female fertility falls naturally with age, especially over the age of 40.

Treatment Specialist treatment can help, but the availability of NHS treatment for 'older' women is limited – mainly because the success rates for 'assisted conception' declines dramatically after the age of 40.

Some other medical problems
Very rarely, some serious illness, such as kidney failure or severe hormone problems, can cause problems with fertility.

Treatment These illnesses will tend to make your periods scanty or absent and are likely to show themselves with a number of other symptoms before causing infertility. It's very unlikely that you'll have one of these illnesses – but if you're concerned, see your GP.

| # Itchy scalp

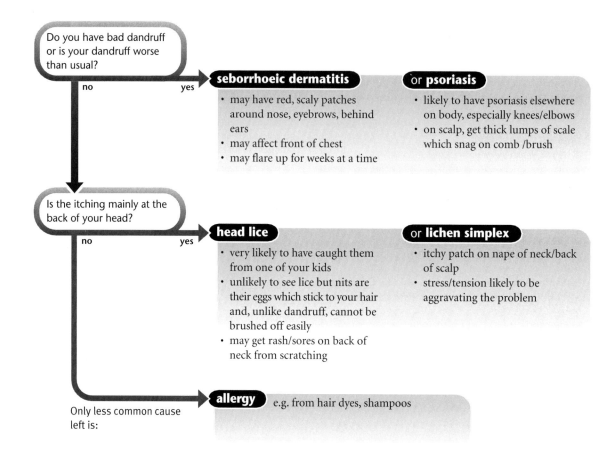

Do you have bad dandruff or is your dandruff worse than usual?

no   **yes**

seborrhoeic dermatitis

- may have red, scaly patches around nose, eyebrows, behind ears
- may affect front of chest
- may flare up for weeks at a time

or psoriasis

- likely to have psoriasis elsewhere on body, especially knees/elbows
- on scalp, get thick lumps of scale which snag on comb /brush

Is the itching mainly at the back of your head?

no   **yes**

head lice

- very likely to have caught them from one of your kids
- unlikely to see lice but nits are their eggs which stick to your hair and, unlike dandruff, cannot be brushed off easily
- may get rash/sores on back of neck from scratching

or lichen simplex

- itchy patch on nape of neck/back of scalp
- stress/tension likely to be aggravating the problem

Only less common cause left is:

allergy   e.g. from hair dyes, shampoos

Itchy scalp

Seborrhoeic dermatitis This is a type of eczema of the scalp caused by an infection with a fungus, which makes the scalp dry, flaky, itchy, and sometimes sore. Dandruff is caused by seborrhoeic dermatitis, which, if mild, leads to some flaking of the scalp but little, if any, itch.

Treatment If you've just got mild dandruff, regular hair washing with an anti-dandruff or anti-fungal shampoo should sort it out. Coal tar-based shampoos are good for the itching but won't get rid of the underlying problem. If you're having terrible problems with dandruff and irritation, see your GP – she can prescribe very effective anti-fungal and anti-itch shampoos and lotions. Seborrhoeic dermatitis can keep coming back, so you may need to repeat the treatment from time to time.

Psoriasis This can affect various parts of the body, including the scalp. It produces a patchy, scaly rash that sometimes gets itchy. On the scalp, the skin gets very thick and roughened, leading to bad dandruff. The cause is unknown, but it sometimes runs in families.

Treatment Strong coal tar shampoos (available from the chemist) can help. Otherwise, you'll need to discuss the situation with your GP, who can prescribe various shampoos or lotions to ease the problem. It can be difficult to sort out and you may need to try a lot of different treatments before you strike lucky – and, like seborrhoeic dermatitis, it can keep coming back. If you have really severe scalp psoriasis and nothing seems to help, your GP may refer you to a dermatologist (skin specialist).

Head lice Lice are tiny insects which can live in your hair – the severe itch is caused by the bites they inflict on your scalp as they suck blood. The problem is much commoner in children but can occur in adults and is passed on by close contact or by sharing brushes or combs. Another type of louse (often called 'crabs') prefers your pubic hair – this one is usually passed on by having sex with an infected partner.

Treatment Get an anti-lice lotion and/or bug-busting comb from the chemist and follow the instructions very closely. And make sure you check your household contacts for lice too, otherwise you'll get infected again (look for nits, which are tiny lice eggs attached near the base of hairs, especially behind the ears – you can tell they're not dandruff because they're quite hard to separate from the hairs). If you've got crabs, apply a lotion from the chemist to your pubic hairs. Check other hairy areas too, as the lice can spread, even to eyebrows and eyelashes; and, of course, enquire delicately whether or not your partner has noticed any wildlife crawling around his undergrowth.

Lichen simplex This is an itchy patch usually found on the nape of the neck and the back of the scalp. It's probably caused by stress: being tense makes you scratch or rub the back of your head, which inflames the skin and which, in turn, causes itching and so more scratching – and so it continues.

Treatment Coal tar shampoos and hydrocortisone 1% cream from the chemist can help relieve the irritation – or you may need something stronger from your GP. But you won't cure the problem unless you stop scratching or rubbing the affected area. Try to sort out whatever's stressing you and check out some of the relaxation measures discussed in the 'Feeling tense' section (p. 64).

Allergy Occasionally, your scalp can get inflamed because of an allergy to something you've put on it. The likeliest culprits are hair dyes and shampoos.

Treatment The problem will sort itself out in a couple of days. Make sure you avoid whatever's brought it on in future.

Itchy skin

N.B. Pregnancy (particularly later on) can cause itching/rashes (see opposite page).

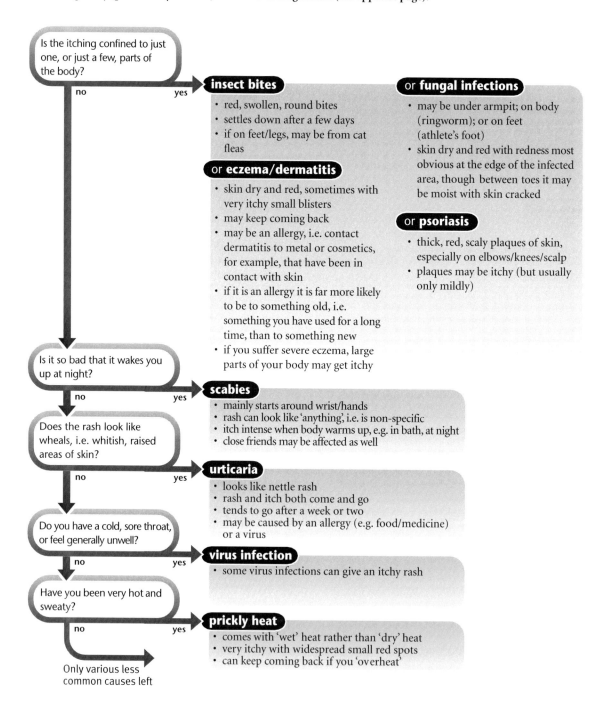

Is the itching confined to just one, or just a few, parts of the body?

no / yes

insect bites
- red, swollen, round bites
- settles down after a few days
- if on feet/legs, may be from cat fleas

or eczema/dermatitis
- skin dry and red, sometimes with very itchy small blisters
- may keep coming back
- may be an allergy, i.e. contact dermatitis to metal or cosmetics, for example, that have been in contact with skin
- if it is an allergy it is far more likely to be to something old, i.e. something you have used for a long time, than to something new
- if you suffer severe eczema, large parts of your body may get itchy

or fungal infections
- may be under armpit; on body (ringworm); or on feet (athlete's foot)
- skin dry and red with redness most obvious at the edge of the infected area, though between toes it may be moist with skin cracked

or psoriasis
- thick, red, scaly plaques of skin, especially on elbows/knees/scalp
- plaques may be itchy (but usually only mildly)

Is it so bad that it wakes you up at night?

no / yes

scabies
- mainly starts around wrist/hands
- rash can look like 'anything', i.e. is non-specific
- itch intense when body warms up, e.g. in bath, at night
- close friends may be affected as well

Does the rash look like wheals, i.e. whitish, raised areas of skin?

no / yes

urticaria
- looks like nettle rash
- rash and itch both come and go
- tends to go after a week or two
- may be caused by an allergy (e.g. food/medicine) or a virus

Do you have a cold, sore throat, or feel generally unwell?

no / yes

virus infection
- some virus infections can give an itchy rash

Have you been very hot and sweaty?

no / yes

prickly heat
- comes with 'wet' heat rather than 'dry' heat
- very itchy with widespread small red spots
- can keep coming back if you 'overheat'

Only various less common causes left

Insect bites Bites from insects produce a characteristic itchy rash.

Treatment Calamine lotion and antihistamine tablets (like you'd use for hay fever – available from the chemist) will ease the problem. And if you have a cat or dog at home, get it checked for fleas.

Eczema/dermatitis This means inflamed skin – it becomes red, itchy, and dry or weepy. There are many different types, each with characteristic patterns. In most cases, the cause is unknown, but a few result from allergy (such as an allergy to the nickel in your jeans buckle or your metal watch strap – but almost never an allergy to something you've eaten). Some start in childhood (especially the type which is linked with hay fever and asthma) and others only appear when you're older.

Treatment This is pretty much the same whatever your type of eczema. First of all, look after your skin: wash regularly but avoid perfumed soaps or bubble baths, and, if your hands are affected, keep them out of detergents – if you must do the washing up, wear rubber gloves (make sure they've got a cotton lining because rubber can aggravate the problem). Moisturizer is important if your skin is dry. You can get various types from the chemist (such as aqueous cream); some people use this as a soap substitute too. It's also worth using a mild steroid cream – hydrocortisone 1% is available over the counter and is perfectly safe to use, even on the face. Bear in mind that these treatments only ease, rather than cure, the problem – unfortunately, eczema can keep coming back, and it's just a case of using the treatments whenever it flares up. Don't mess around with your diet, either, as this almost never helps. If the pattern of your eczema suggests an allergy then avoid whatever you think might be bringing it on. And if you've tried all the measures described without much effect, see your GP – she'll be able to prescribe you other treatments to get on top of the problem.

Scabies This is caused by a microscopic insect which burrows into the skin. The rash is actually an allergy to the insect's droppings, and can be incredibly itchy. It is passed on by close contact but may take a few weeks to develop.

Treatment You can get anti-scabies lotions from the chemist. It's vital that you read the instructions carefully and apply it exactly as directed, otherwise it won't work. Make sure close contacts (such as family and partner) are treated too. The itch can take a few weeks to go away. Don't make the mistake of thinking the treatment hasn't worked – if you keep putting on the lotion, you'll just irritate the skin more.

Urticaria Also known as hives or nettle rash. It's usually caused by an allergy to something you've eaten (like nuts, shellfish, or strawberries) or to a medicine (such as an antibiotic). It can also be brought on by viruses and some other rare illnesses. Another type of urticaria, which can keep coming back, can be caused by the skin being irritated by pressure or contact with water.

Treatment Use calamine lotion and antihistamine tablets (see above). If it turns out to be an allergy, avoid the offending food or medicine in the future.

Fungal infections See the 'Rash' section (p. 126).

Virus See the 'Rash' section (p. 126). Some viruses – especially chickenpox – can result in rashes which are quite itchy (chickenpox is discussed further in the 'Blisters' section, p. 30).

Prickly heat This rash, which can be extremely itchy, appears on areas exposed to the sun. The cause is unknown, but it tends to keep coming back for a few years whenever you go out in the sun in the summer, before it eventually fizzles out.

Treatment The usual calamine lotion and antihistamine tablet routine may help. Stay out of the sun as much as possible, keep cool, and wash the skin regularly.

Psoriasis This is explained, and its treatment outlined, in the 'Rash' section (p. 126). It can sometimes cause itching.

Pregnancy Very itchy skin problems (some with a rash and some without) can be caused by the hormone changes that occur in pregnancy.

Treatment It's usually just a case of using moisturizers or calamine lotion to ease the problem, which will go once you've had the baby. If the skin is very itchy, you'll need to see your GP to confirm the cause; you might need blood tests or, very rarely, treatment by a dermatologist. Some of these problems come back in future pregnancies and some don't – your doctor should be able to advise you.

Other less common causes These include other skin diseases (like lichen planus, which causes itchy marks on the wrists, arms, and legs); certain illnesses (such as diabetes and kidney disease) which can make the skin itch without a rash; psychological problems (stress can set up a vicious cycle of scratching the skin, causing irritation, leading to itching, resulting in further irritation); and the side-effects of medication.

Treatment If you think you have one of these problems, discuss it with your GP.

Knee pain

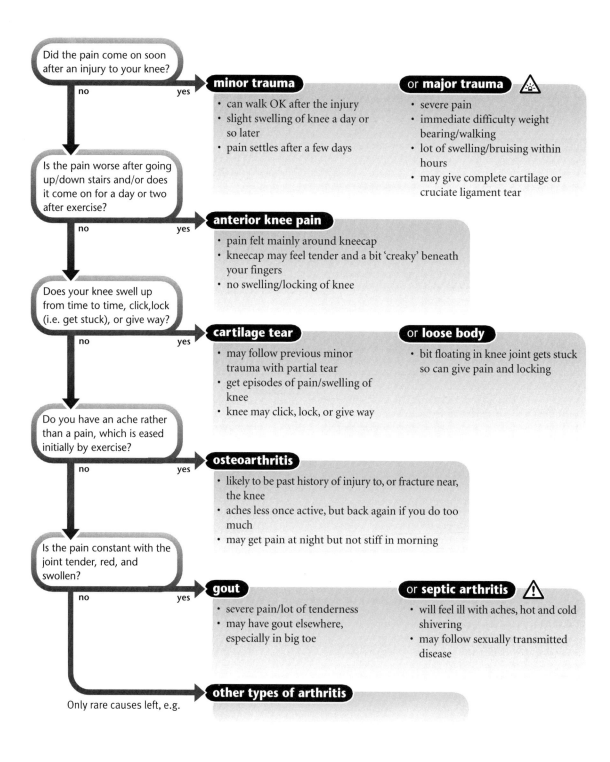

Did the pain come on soon after an injury to your knee?

no / yes

minor trauma
- can walk OK after the injury
- slight swelling of knee a day or so later
- pain settles after a few days

or major trauma
- severe pain
- immediate difficulty weight bearing/walking
- lot of swelling/bruising within hours
- may give complete cartilage or cruciate ligament tear

Is the pain worse after going up/down stairs and/or does it come on for a day or two after exercise?

no / yes

anterior knee pain
- pain felt mainly around kneecap
- kneecap may feel tender and a bit 'creaky' beneath your fingers
- no swelling/locking of knee

Does your knee swell up from time to time, click,lock (i.e. get stuck), or give way?

no / yes

cartilage tear
- may follow previous minor trauma with partial tear
- get episodes of pain/swelling of knee
- knee may click, lock, or give way

or loose body
- bit floating in knee joint gets stuck so can give pain and locking

Do you have an ache rather than a pain, which is eased initially by exercise?

no / yes

osteoarthritis
- likely to be past history of injury to, or fracture near, the knee
- aches less once active, but back again if you do too much
- may get pain at night but not stiff in morning

Is the pain constant with the joint tender, red, and swollen?

no / yes

gout
- severe pain/lot of tenderness
- may have gout elsewhere, especially in big toe

or septic arthritis
- will feel ill with aches, hot and cold shivering
- may follow sexually transmitted disease

other types of arthritis

Only rare causes left, e.g.

Minor trauma A mild bump or twist of the knee can cause bruising or a sprain of a ligament (the tough cords holding the knees together). Sometimes, after an injury, the lining of the joint gets inflamed and leaks some fluid, causing slight swelling of the knee a day or so afterwards.

Treatment Remember 'RICE', especially if the knee swells a little: Rest, Ice, Compression, and Elevation. So you should rest the knee for a day or two (elevated on a stool), put an ice-pack on it (like a bag of frozen peas wrapped in a flannel), and use a firm bandage. After a couple of days, the pain should settle – a painkiller may help too (particularly an anti-inflammatory like ibuprofen, which is available from the chemist). Once things are improving, keep the knee strong with quadriceps exercises – the quadriceps are the muscles of the thigh and you can exercise them by putting a weight on your feet and repeatedly straightening out your legs. When you feel confident, get back to your normal activities, including sport – but break yourself back in gently and don't forget to warm up. If you keep getting trouble, see your GP: she might suggest some further treatment such as physiotherapy.

Anterior knee pain This simply means repeated pain in the front of the knee. It's usually caused by a roughening of the underneath of the kneecap or by the thigh muscles inflaming the areas of bone they pull on.

Treatment This usually goes away on its own, although it can take months. If you do a lot of running, try more gentle exercise (like swimming) for a while before gradually getting back into your normal routine. Avoid forcibly bending the knees too much – so keep squatting or kneeling to a minimum. And if you do a lot of cycling, make sure your saddle is high enough to make your legs straighten out when you pedal. Quadriceps exercises and anti-inflammatory pills (as above) may help.

Torn cartilage The cartilage is the knee's shock absorber – it can be torn by a twisting injury.

Treatment A very minor tear may settle with the advice given above for minor trauma. Otherwise, see your GP, who is likely to refer you to an orthopaedic surgeon (bone specialist).

Osteoarthritis When your knee cartilage gradually wears down, the bones tend to grind over each other, causing a repeated ache – this is osteoarthritis. It's particularly common if you are overweight, have had a serious injury or

operation to your knee, or if your knees have suffered through work or sport.

Treatment Painkillers, anti-inflammatories, and quads exercises, as already outlined, are helpful. If you're overweight, try to slim down. Continue exercising, as this keeps the joints supple and the muscles strong – but gentle exercise, like swimming, is much better than anything which jars, such as jogging. You may find that wearing spongy soles, or putting a thick sponge insole into your shoes, acts as a shock absorber, relieving the pressure on your knees. If you're getting nowhere, talk to your GP – but don't expect an X-ray, as this doesn't usually help much. Surgery can cure very arthritic knees, but this is usually reserved for the elderly who are badly disabled by the problem.

Loose body A flake of bone or cartilage can float around in the joint. These 'loose bodies' are often the result of a previous injury.

Treatment This is a job for an orthopaedic specialist if the symptoms are a real nuisance – so speak to your GP, who will probably arrange an appointment for you.

Major trauma A serious knee injury – for example in a road accident, or through skiing – can cause a broken bone or a complete tear of a large ligament (such as the 'ruptured cruciate' – a tear of the main ligaments of the knee). The pain is obviously severe and is usually quickly followed – within an hour or so – by dramatic swelling.

Treatment Go straight to casualty.

Gout This is covered in the 'Pain in the ankle, foot, or toe' section (p. 110). The knee is the second commonest site for this to happen, after the big toe.

Septic arthritis This is an infection caused by a germ entering the joint. It's sometimes caused by an infected wound, or, very occasionally, by a sexually transmitted bug entering the bloodstream and ending up in the joint.

Treatment See your GP asap – she is likely to admit you to hospital for powerful antibiotic treatment.

Other forms of arthritis There are a number of types of joint diseases (such as rheumatoid arthritis) which can affect the knee, but they are all quite unusual.

Treatment If you think you have this type of problem, see your GP – if she agrees, you're likely to be referred to a rheumatologist (joint specialist).

Loss of consciousness

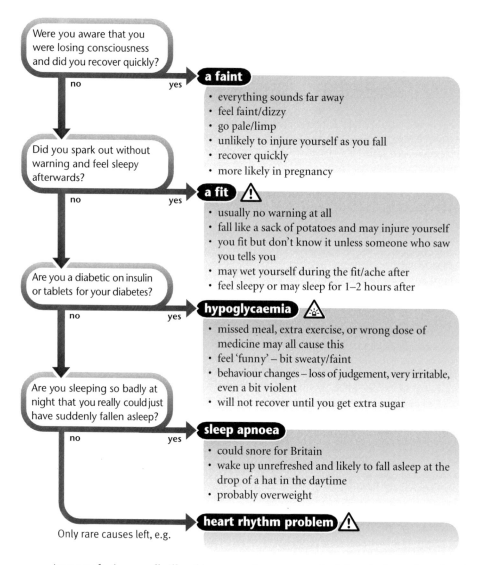

Were you aware that you were losing consciousness and did you recover quickly?

no — yes

a faint
- everything sounds far away
- feel faint/dizzy
- go pale/limp
- unlikely to injure yourself as you fall
- recover quickly
- more likely in pregnancy

Did you spark out without warning and feel sleepy afterwards?

no — yes

a fit ⚠
- usually no warning at all
- fall like a sack of potatoes and may injure yourself
- you fit but don't know it unless someone who saw you tells you
- may wet yourself during the fit/ache after
- feel sleepy or may sleep for 1–2 hours after

Are you a diabetic on insulin or tablets for your diabetes?

no — yes

hypoglycaemia ⚠
- missed meal, extra exercise, or wrong dose of medicine may all cause this
- feel 'funny' – bit sweaty/faint
- behaviour changes – loss of judgement, very irritable, even a bit violent
- will not recover until you get extra sugar

Are you sleeping so badly at night that you really could just have suddenly fallen asleep?

no — yes

sleep apnoea
- could snore for Britain
- wake up unrefreshed and likely to fall asleep at the drop of a hat in the daytime
- probably overweight

heart rhythm problem ⚠

Only rare causes left, e.g.

⚠ Anyone who is generally ill and loses consciousness, or who is knocked out after a head injury, should be taken straight to hospital.

Remember: ⚠ means see your GP sharpish; ⚠ means an urgent hospital job

Loss of consciousness

A faint If not enough blood is getting to your brain, you'll pass out – this is nature's way of solving the problem, because you end up horizontal so that your blood isn't having to go uphill anymore to your oxygen-starved brain. A variety of things can trigger a faint. The most typical is standing for a long time somewhere hot and stuffy: normally, your leg movements pump blood back into the circulation, but if you've been standing still for a while, particularly anywhere hot, your blood will 'pool' in your legs, causing a faint. Jumping up quickly out of a hot bath can have the same effect. Other causes include pregnancy, a severe spasm of coughing (which prevents the blood getting to the brain), and sudden fear or pain (which slow the heart rate). Being a bit run down – such as when you have the flu – can also make you more likely to faint. Some people just seem prone to faints and get a number of attacks, but this is almost never caused by any serious disease. Certain medications (such as some blood pressure pills and antidepressants) can also cause faints or near faints.

Treatment The treatment of someone who is fainting is quite simple – catch her, if you're quick enough, so she doesn't injure herself, then gently lay her down. Raise her feet about 30 degrees in the air, as this will help drain blood back to her brain so that she should recover in a few seconds. If you feel as though you're going to faint, lie down as soon as you can; if this is impossible, sit down with your head between your knees until the feeling has passed. People who are prone to fainting can help prevent attacks by avoiding trigger situations and pumping their calf muscles (by moving their feet up and down as if using an invisible accelerator) if they've been standing still for a while. If you're on prescribed treatment which you think might be causing or aggravating the problem, speak to your GP.

A fit The easiest way to understand a fit is to imagine that the various nerve connections in the brain are like a complex system of electrical wires. A short circuit in this system can result in a variety of types of fit. The most well known is the 'grand mal fit' but there are many other sorts, and some of them can be quite subtle. What causes fits is unknown, although the problem sometimes runs in families. There are a number of things that can trigger fits, including extreme tiredness, an alcoholic binge, flashing lights and, in a known epileptic, forgetting to take your tablets.

Treatment If you think you've had a fit – or someone who was with you at the time reckons that was what happened – make an appointment to see your GP. Try to take someone who can give an eyewitness account, as you'll only be aware

of the events leading up to, and immediately after, passing out. Your GP will refer you to a neurologist (nervous system specialist) for further tests. You're unlikely immediately to be labelled as 'epileptic' as many people suffer just one fit and never have another. If you do get further fits though, you're likely to be told you have epilepsy and you'll be put on treatment to try to keep future fits to a minimum. Remember to inform the DVLA (Driver and Licensing Agency) and your car insurers if you develop this problem – you may be banned from driving for a year or more, depending on the circumstances.

Hypoglycaemia This means a low blood sugar level, which effectively starves the brain of energy. If this is the cause of your loss of consciousness, you either have some very rare illness or you're a diabetic. Diabetics on treatment are very prone to this problem, usually because of a missed meal, an unusual amount of exercise, or incorrect doses of diabetic tablets or insulin.

Treatment You need sugar asap. If you're just about conscious enough to swallow then hopefully someone will be forcing a sweet drink down you. But if not, you'll be carted off to hospital for treatment. When you've recovered, try to figure out why it happened. If your sugars have been running low for a while, it may be that your diabetes treatment needs altering. Discuss this with your GP or the local diabetic nurse if you're not confident in making any changes yourself.

Sleep apnoea Loads of people snore badly at night. In a few, the snoring can actually make the breathing stop from time to time. This is sleep apnoea. You won't be aware of this, but your partner will, because he'll be lying awake at night wondering if you've just gasped your last. This problem tends to disturb your sleep and can make you so tired that you tend to drop off ridiculously easily during the day – for example, during a meal or while driving.

Treatment If you're overweight, slim down and avoid alcoholic nightcaps. But if this doesn't sort it out, see your GP, and take your partner with you so he can give her an ear-witness account. You're likely to be referred to an Ear, Nose, and Throat ('ENT') specialist if it's causing real problems.

Rare medical causes There are a few small-print causes of loss of consciousness, such as heart rhythm or valve problems. They are all very unusual and are likely to produce a variety of other symptoms to give the game away.

Treatment If your GP suspects a rare cause like this, she'll refer you to a specialist for tests.

Loss of sex drive

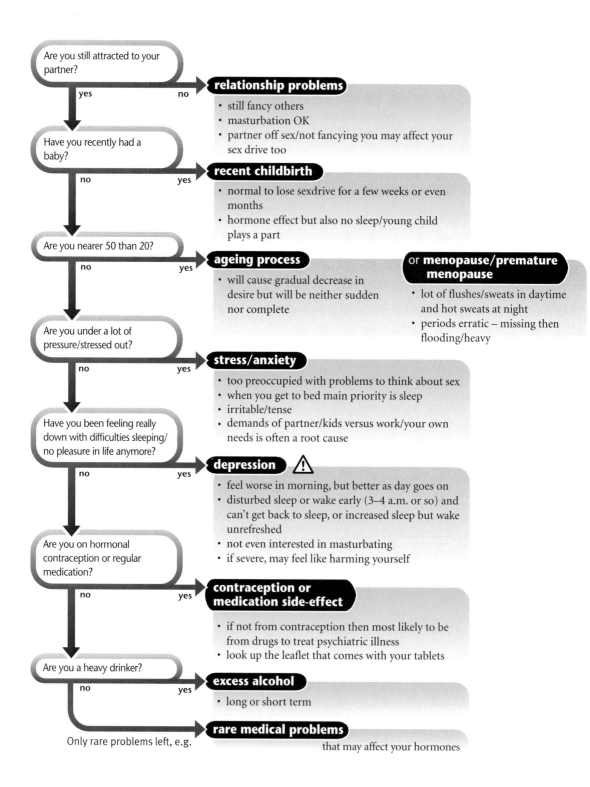

relationship problems
- still fancy others
- masturbation OK
- partner off sex/not fancying you may affect your sex drive too

recent childbirth
- normal to lose sexdrive for a few weeks or even months
- hormone effect but also no sleep/young child plays a part

ageing process
- will cause gradual decrease in desire but will be neither sudden nor complete

or menopause/premature menopause
- lot of flushes/sweats in daytime and hot sweats at night
- periods erratic – missing then flooding/heavy

stress/anxiety
- too preoccupied with problems to think about sex
- when you get to bed main priority is sleep
- irritable/tense
- demands of partner/kids versus work/your own needs is often a root cause

depression ⚠
- feel worse in morning, but better as day goes on
- disturbed sleep or wake early (3–4 a.m. or so) and can't get back to sleep, or increased sleep but wake unrefreshed
- not even interested in masturbating
- if severe, may feel like harming yourself

contraception or medication side-effect
- if not from contraception then most likely to be from drugs to treat psychiatric illness
- look up the leaflet that comes with your tablets

excess alcohol
- long or short term

rare medical problems

Only rare problems left, e.g. that may affect your hormones

Stress/anxiety You may simply be too worried about a whole load of problems and stresses to have time to think about sex. And then, as the saying goes, if you don't use it, you lose it – you can fall into the habit of not having sex, and this develops into a lack of interest. Anxiety can affect your sex drive in other ways. For example, you may be worried about getting (or not getting) pregnant, or you might be concerned that you're not performing well in bed. Worries like this – and fear of failure in particular – can end up turning you off sex, because this is a way of avoiding the situation.

Treatment If you're generally feeling tense, look at the advice in the 'Lifestyle/stress' part of the 'Feeling tense' section (p. 64). Try to discuss the situation with your partner, he's bound to have noticed that you've gone off sex, and will probably be worried about the situation too, so it's best to get it out in the open. If the problem doesn't improve, consider seeing your GP – and try to get your partner to go with you. Your GP herself may be able to help, or she may refer you to a psychosexual counsellor (an expert in talking through these problems who can try to help you solve them).

Relationship problems It's not surprising that if you're having constant rows with your partner, or you've simply gone off each other, then your sex life will suffer. Unless the stress is really getting to you, you'll probably still have some sex drive – it just won't be directed towards your partner.

Treatment There's obviously no magic answer to this one other than to try to sort out the problem with your partner.

Recent childbirth Most couples find their sex life goes off the boil for a few weeks – or even months – after the arrival of a baby. There are a number of reasons for this, including hormone changes, sheer knackeredness, and your change of role. And your partner may be sulking because of the attention the baby's getting or might find breast feeding a bit of a turn-off.

Treatment This should correct itself given time. Try to discuss the situation with your partner, otherwise any simmering tensions or frustrations will tend to aggrevate the problem.

Depression Your sex drive is one of many areas that depression can affect. It is explained further, and its treatment outlined, in the 'Feeling down' section (p. 62).

Ageing It's quite normal for your sex drive to fluctuate and fall as you get older. This is partly due to the ageing process itself but also to relationship problems, stress and overwork.

Treatment There is no magic pill for this. Try to sort out problem areas that are in your control. If your decreased sex drive is causing problems with your partner try to discuss things openly and sort them out together.

Menopause/premature menopause The hormone changes which happen around the time of the menopause can affect your sex drive. For more details, see the 'Flushing' section (p. 66).

Medication side-effect The Pill can sometimes lower sex drive. This is quite unusual – the Pill is often blamed as the cause when there's actually some other cause, such as a relationship problem. Some other prescribed medication can lower sex drive – for example, it can occur with some drugs used to treat psychiatric conditions. In these cases, it's difficult to know if the problem is an effect of the drug or an effect of the illness the drug is being used to treat.

Treatment If you feel reasonably certain that the Pill really is the cause of the problem then speak to you GP about switching to another type of pill or an alternative family planning method. You should also speak to your GP if you're on some medication which you think could be affecting your sex life.

Alcohol In the short term, after a binge, you may simply be too tiddly to care about sex. In the long term too much alcohol can cause damage to your physical and emotional health. Loss of sex drive will be just one of many problems you are likely to experience.

Treatment Cut down the booze and don't binge. If your loss of sex drive is caused by alcoholism you're obviously in serious trouble and need to see your GP or seek other professional help.

Rare medical problems Various unusual illnesses, particularly those which affect hormones, can lower your sex drive.

Treatment It's highly unlikely that you'll have any of these medical rarities. If you're concerned, see your GP, who will check out the problem.

Lower abdominal pain – one-off

N.B. Specific pregnancy (more than 12 weeks' gestation) causes of abdominal pain are not covered. If you are pregnant and your pain is not obviously caused by cystitis or gastroenteritis, then seek medical advice quickly.

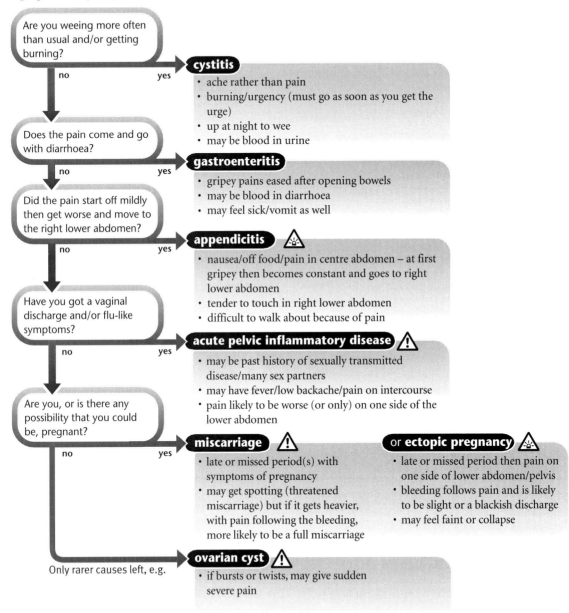

Are you weeing more often than usual and/or getting burning? — no / yes

cystitis
- ache rather than pain
- burning/urgency (must go as soon as you get the urge)
- up at night to wee
- may be blood in urine

Does the pain come and go with diarrhoea? — no / yes

gastroenteritis
- gripey pains eased after opening bowels
- may be blood in diarrhoea
- may feel sick/vomit as well

Did the pain start off mildly then get worse and move to the right lower abdomen? — no / yes

appendicitis
- nausea/off food/pain in centre abdomen – at first gripey then becomes constant and goes to right lower abdomen
- tender to touch in right lower abdomen
- difficult to walk about because of pain

Have you got a vaginal discharge and/or flu-like symptoms? — no / yes

acute pelvic inflammatory disease
- may be past history of sexually transmitted disease/many sex partners
- may have fever/low backache/pain on intercourse
- pain likely to be worse (or only) on one side of the lower abdomen

Are you, or is there any possibility that you could be, pregnant? — no / yes

miscarriage
- late or missed period(s) with symptoms of pregnancy
- may get spotting (threatened miscarriage) but if it gets heavier, with pain following the bleeding, more likely to be a full miscarriage

or ectopic pregnancy
- late or missed period then pain on one side of lower abdomen/pelvis
- bleeding follows pain and is likely to be slight or a blackish discharge
- may feel faint or collapse

Only rarer causes left, e.g.

ovarian cyst
- if bursts or twists, may give sudden severe pain

 If your abdominal pain is severe, or you feel ill or faint with it, then the actual diagnosis does not matter – it is likely to have a serious cause and you must seek medical attention immediately.

Cystitis This is explained, and the treatment discussed, in the 'Waterworks problems' section (p. 160). The bladder – the muscular bag which collects your urine – is low down in your abdomen so, when inflamed by an infection, it can cause a lower abdominal ache.

Gastroenteritis This is explained, and its treatment outlined, in the 'Abdominal pain – one-off' section (p.8).

Miscarriage This is explained, and the treatment discussed, in the 'Miscarriage/threatened miscarriage' part of the 'Abdominal or irregular vaginal bleeding' section (p. 16).

Appendicitis This is discussed in the 'Abdominal pain – one-off' section (p. 8).

Acute pelvic inflammatory disease The pelvic organs – the womb, ovaries, and the tubes connecting these parts together (the fallopian tubes) – can sometimes become infected with germs. These infections may be caused by a sexually transmitted infection (such as chlamidia or gonorrhoea) or the germs may get into your pelvic organs some other way – for example, through having recently had a baby, an abortion, or a coil fitted. They cause inflammation ('acute pelvic inflammatory disease') which results in pain and, possibly, abnormal bleeding or discharge from the vagina too. Sometimes, the infection 'sets in', causing repeated attacks, heavy periods and, in some cases, fertility problems (see the 'Heavy periods' section, p. 72).

Treatment You need to see your GP urgently. She may be able to solve the problem with antibiotics if it's a mild attack. Otherwise, you'll be sent to hospital – especially if the problem follows childbirth or an abortion, as this means some tissue or blood has probably been left behind, causing the infection. This requires antibiotics and, usually, a 'scrape' – the removal of the tissue under anaesthetic.

Ectopic pregnancy A pregnancy developing outside of the womb – usually in one of the fallopian tubes – is called 'ectopic'. As the pregnancy develops, it stretches the tube, causing pain or a sudden loss of blood. Ectopic pregnancies are sometimes caused by the fallopian tubes being damaged and so are more common in women who've had surgery on, or infections in, their tubes. Pregnancies which occur in women using the coil or taking the progestogen-only pill (the 'mini-pill') are also more likely to be ectopic.

Treatment If you think you might have an ectopic pregnancy then you should seek medical attention without delay, so speak to your GP or go to hospital. You will certainly need to be assessed urgently in hospital if it turns out there is a chance you could have an ectopic, because of the risk it may 'rupture' – in other words, burst the fallopian tube, leading to a lot of blood loss and making you very ill indeed.

Ovarian cyst An ovarian cyst is a lump, often filled with fluid, which develops on your ovary. It can burst ('rupture') or twist, leading to sudden and severe pain.

Treatment Sudden pain caused by an ovarian cyst is a hospital job.

Lower abdominal pain – recurrent

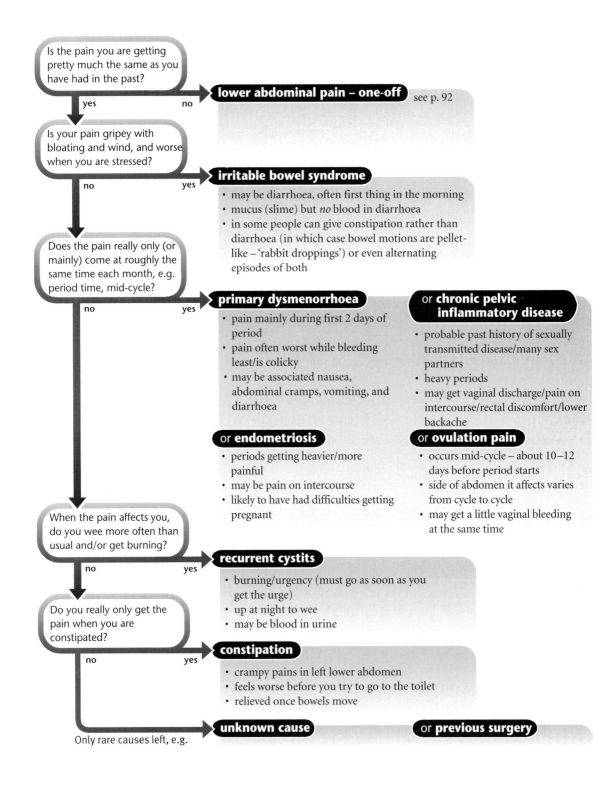

Is the pain you are getting pretty much the same as you have had in the past?

lower abdominal pain – one-off see p. 92

yes / no

Is your pain gripey with bloating and wind, and worse when you are stressed?

no / yes

irritable bowel syndrome
- may be diarrhoea, often first thing in the morning
- mucus (slime) but *no* blood in diarrhoea
- in some people can give constipation rather than diarrhoea (in which case bowel motions are pellet-like – 'rabbit droppings') or even alternating episodes of both

Does the pain really only (or mainly) come at roughly the same time each month, e.g. period time, mid-cycle?

no / yes

primary dysmenorrhoea
- pain mainly during first 2 days of period
- pain often worst while bleeding least/is colicky
- may be associated nausea, abdominal cramps, vomiting, and diarrhoea

or **chronic pelvic inflammatory disease**
- probable past history of sexually transmitted disease/many sex partners
- heavy periods
- may get vaginal discharge/pain on intercourse/rectal discomfort/lower backache

or **endometriosis**
- periods getting heavier/more painful
- may be pain on intercourse
- likely to have had difficulties getting pregnant

or **ovulation pain**
- occurs mid-cycle – about 10–12 days before period starts
- side of abdomen it affects varies from cycle to cycle
- may get a little vaginal bleeding at the same time

When the pain affects you, do you wee more often than usual and/or get burning?

no / yes

recurrent cystits
- burning/urgency (must go as soon as you get the urge)
- up at night to wee
- may be blood in urine

Do you really only get the pain when you are constipated?

no / yes

constipation
- crampy pains in left lower abdomen
- feels worse before you try to go to the toilet
- relieved once bowels move

unknown cause or **previous surgery**

Only rare causes left, e.g.

Lower abdominal pain – recurrent

Primary dysmenorrhoea This is simply medical jargon for 'normal' period pains. See 'Painful periods' section (p. 114).

Irritable bowel syndrome This is explained, in the 'Abdominal pains – recurrent' section (p. 10).

Chronic pelvic inflammatory disease The pelvic organs – the womb, ovaries, and the tubes connecting these parts together (the fallopian tubes) – can sometimes become infected with germs which fail to disappear on their own or even after antibiotic treatment. They cause inflammation which, in turn, leads to repeated episodes of pain (and, often, heavy periods).

Treatment See your GP. Repeated or long courses of antibiotics sometimes help, or she may refer you to a gynaecologist for possible surgery, particularly if the inflammation has led to swelling of your fallopian tubes.

Endometriosis The lining of the womb (the 'endometrium') appears in unexpected places – such as on the ovary, on the ligaments which support the womb, or in the muscular wall of the womb. The precise cause is unknown. It can cause infertility and heavy periods, as well as lower abdominal pain.

Treatment One problem is that it affects different women in different ways. Some appear to have terrible endometriosis yet have few or no symptoms; others have only minor areas of disease yet suffer very badly. So a diagnosis does not necessarily mean that it is the cause of your particular symptom – which is probably why the results of the treatment can sometimes seem disappointing. A definite diagnosis requires hospital tests, so treatment you receive will probably be arranged by the gynaecologist your GP referred you to – it usually consists of hormone tablets or injections, or sometimes surgery.

Ovulation pain When the 'egg' is released from your ovary, around the middle of your cycle, you may experience some mild pain in your lower abdomen.

Treatment This is quite normal. A simple painkiller like paracetamol is usually adequate. The Pill can help, as this prevents the egg being released, although it would be unusual for ovulation pain to be bad enough to need this type of treatment.

Recurrent cystitis See the 'Waterworks problems' section (p. 160).

Constipation If the bowel gets overloaded because you're not going to the toilet regularly, you are likely to feel vaguely uncomfortable most of the time – and suffer bouts of colicky pains as the bowel tries to squeeze stuff through.

Treatment Increase your fibre and fluid intake. Physical exercise helps too. Some medicines – especially painkillers – can cause constipation, so if you take something regularly, check with the chemist to see if it's the culprit. And if all else fails, think about using one of the multitude of over-the-counter laxatives – though just for a few days – to kick-start your bowel.

Previous surgery Previous operations (on the abdomen or pelvic organs) can cause problems that result in repeated bouts of abdominal pain. One example is 'adhesions': organs in the abdomen and pelvis which have been handled during surgery can develop sticky areas which glue to nearby structures, resulting in attacks of pain. Another is 'trapped ovary syndrome', in which surgery results in an ovary getting stuck to tissue at the top of the vagina.

Treatment Straightforward adhesions are best treated with simple painkillers. Further surgery can be attempted to 'free up' the area, but there is a danger of this making matters worse. Trapped ovary syndrome usually requires an operation, so if your GP thinks this might be the problem, she's likely to refer you back to your gynaecologist.

Unknown cause Unfortunately, some women seem to experience repeated lower abdominal pain for which a cause remains elusive and which is very difficult to treat. Doctors sometime call this 'chronic pelvic pain'. Women with this problem end up seeing a number of GPs and gynaecologists, and undergoing several often unpleasant tests in the search for an answer. Sometimes, doctors will find an abnormality – such as a small area of endometriosis (see above) – which seems to explain the problem. But then, typically, it turns out to be a red herring, as appropriate treatment makes no difference. It's perhaps not surprising that women with pelvic pain may suffer depression. In some cases, it may be the cause of the problem and in others, the result of the pain and the frustration. Psychological upsets may play a role another way, as some women with unexplained pelvic pain have suffered a previous emotional trauma, such as sexual abuse, which may be the underlying cause of the problem.

Treatment This is obviously very difficult when the precise cause isn't clear. If you've been thoroughly checked over by gynaecologists and no specific problem has been found, then your GP may be reluctant to send you for more tests. She may want to explore the psychological aspects of your illness. Try to aproach this with an open mind. After all, if you *have* become depressed, it doesn't matter whether it's the cause or the result of your pain.

Rare causes Cysts (lumps on the ovary, often filled with fluid) or even cancers (of the ovary, womb, or bowel) may very occasionally cause recurrent lower abdominal pain.

Treatment These problems are unlikely to be the result of your symptoms. If you're concerned, you should discuss the situation with your GP.

Lumps in the back passage

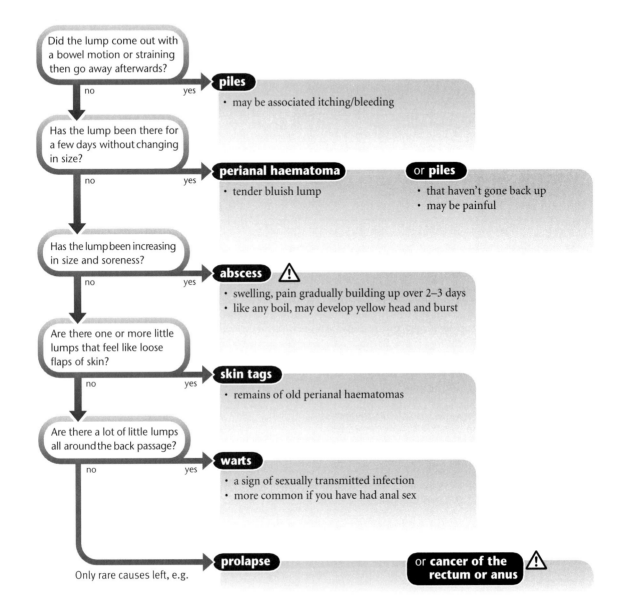

Did the lump come out with a bowel motion or straining then go away afterwards?
   no   yes

piles
• may be associated itching/bleeding

Has the lump been there for a few days without changing in size?
   no   yes

perianal haematoma
• tender bluish lump

or piles
• that haven't gone back up
• may be painful

Has the lump been increasing in size and soreness?
   no   yes

abscess ⚠
• swelling, pain gradually building up over 2–3 days
• like any boil, may develop yellow head and burst

Are there one or more little lumps that feel like loose flaps of skin?
   no   yes

skin tags
• remains of old perianal haematomas

Are there a lot of little lumps all around the back passage?
   no   yes

warts
• a sign of sexually transmitted infection
• more common if you have had anal sex

Only rare causes left, e.g.

prolapse

or cancer of the rectum or anus ⚠

Remember: ⚠ means see your GP sharpish; ⚠ means an urgent hospital job

Lumps in the back passage

Perianal haematoma This is explained, and the treatment outlined, in the 'Pain in the bottom' section (p. 112).

Piles These are varicose veins (swollen blood vessels) in the back passage. They are usually caused by constipation making you strain when you go to the toilet – this forces blood into the veins. As the veins get bigger, they develop into lumps which poke out of your bottom when you sit on the toilet. They may go back up inside on their own, or you may have to push them up with your finger. Sometimes, they stay out all the time; if they get throttled ('strangulated') by the ring-muscle of your back passage, they get very painful (see the 'Prolapsed piles' part of the 'Pain in the bottom' section, p. 112). They can also bleed if the veins burst (see the 'Bleeding from the back passage' section, p. 28).

Treatment This is fully explained in the 'Bleeding from the back passage' section (p. 27).

Skin tags These are souvenirs of previous perianal haematomas (see above). The blood inside these lumps slowly dissolves away, but, because it has stretched the skin around the back passage, you tend to be left with a small, loose flap of skin – these are skin tags.

Treatment Skin tags are totally harmless, usually cause no problem whatsoever, and should simply be left alone.

Abscess This is explained, and the treatment discussed, in the 'Pain in the bottom' section (p. 112). The pain will usually appear before you can actually feel a lump.

Warts These are caused by a virus and are usually passed on sexually. They are normaly found around the front passage but can occur around the back passage too – especially if you indulge in anal sex. Their size varies from tiny pimples to fleshy lumps.

Treatment See the 'Vulval irritation and/or sores' section (p. 158).

Other rare causes These include prolapses and cancer of the back passage. A prolapse means something hanging down – in this case, the lining of your back passage. This is nearly always caused by severe straining because of constipation and is very unusual in the under 50s. Thankfully, cancer of the back passage is also very rare.

Treatment To stop a prolapse getting any worse, sort out your constipation. This means high-fibre foods, plenty of fluids, and more physical exercise. If possible, only use laxatives from the chemist if you're desperate, and just for a week or two. A prolapse in itself isn't harmful, but may be uncomfortable and can irritate or bleed. The only cure is surgery, so discuss the situation with your GP if it's becoming a real problem. If you're worried you might have cancer, then obviously it's a GP job – but you're much more likely to get reassurance or a harmless diagnosis like piles than some bad news and an urgent appointment with a bottom specialist.

Mouth ulcers

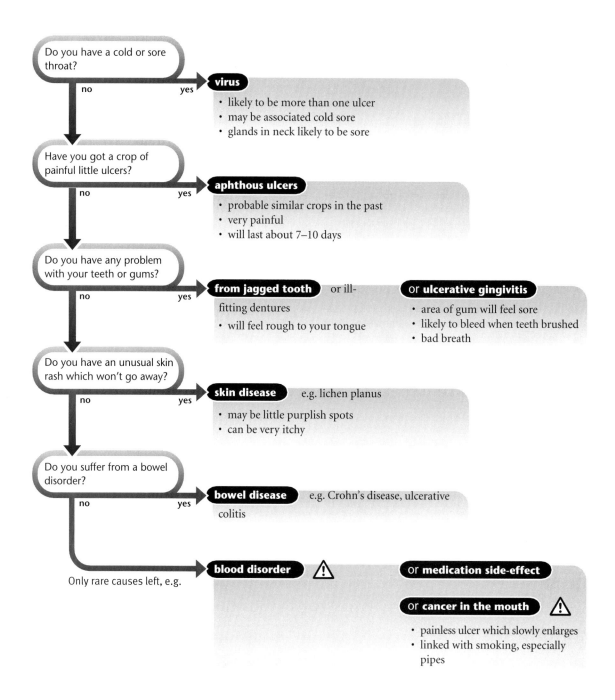

Do you have a cold or sore throat?

no | yes

virus
- likely to be more than one ulcer
- may be associated cold sore
- glands in neck likely to be sore

Have you got a crop of painful little ulcers?

no | yes

aphthous ulcers
- probable similar crops in the past
- very painful
- will last about 7–10 days

Do you have any problem with your teeth or gums?

no | yes

from jagged tooth or ill-fitting dentures
- will feel rough to your tongue

or ulcerative gingivitis
- area of gum will feel sore
- likely to bleed when teeth brushed
- bad breath

Do you have an unusual skin rash which won't go away?

no | yes

skin disease e.g. lichen planus
- may be little purplish spots
- can be very itchy

Do you suffer from a bowel disorder?

no | yes

bowel disease e.g. Crohn's disease, ulcerative colitis

Only rare causes left, e.g.

blood disorder ⚠

or medication side-effect

or cancer in the mouth ⚠
- painless ulcer which slowly enlarges
- linked with smoking, especially pipes

Remember: ⚠ means see your GP sharpish; ⚠ means an urgent hospital job

Aphthous ulcers These are the common mouth ulcers which many people get at times. They are usually very small and may appear in clusters; sometimes, larger single ulcers develop and can take longer to heal. No one knows what causes them, although they sometimes run in families.

Treatment Small ulcers go away on their own in a few days; larger ones can take longer. The chemist will sell you various gels or pastes which may help. As the cause is unknown, there's no real way you can prevent them. It has been suggested that they are a sign of vitamin deficiency, but, in fact, this is hardly ever the case, so vitamin pills almost certainly won't help.

Virus Virus-type germs can cause mouth ulcers among their more familiar symptoms, such as sore throat and fever. For example, a bad attack of the cold sore virus can cause ulcers inside the lips and on the tongue and gums; another virus is known as 'hand, foot, and mouth' because it causes spots on the hands and feet, and ulcers in the mouth (it has nothing to do with the foot and mouth disease of cows).

Treatment As with most viruses, the only treatment is to wait for the body to fight it off – this normally takes seven to 10 days. In the meantime, drink plenty of fluids and take painkillers if necessary.

Trauma from a jagged tooth The sharp edge of a tooth can wear away the surface of the nearby tongue or inner cheek, resulting in an ulcer.

Treatment The ulcer will only clear if the tooth problem is sorted out – so see a dentist.

Ulcerative gingivitis This is an infection of the gums caused by a germ. It is usually linked to neglect of the teeth and gums.

Treatment Another dentist job. Antibiotics will clear the infection, but to prevent future problems the dentist will need to give you a check-up, and you'll have to get working with the brush and floss. Smoking tends to aggravate it too.

Skin disease Some fairly unusual skin diseases can affect the mouth, resulting in ulcers. Occasionally, a disease of this sort causing ulcers leaves the rest of your skin alone, so there may be no skin rashes or blisters to give the game away.

Treatment Discuss the problem with your GP. If you do have skin rashes elsewhere she may be able to piece it all together and treat you, or she may need to refer you to a dermatologist (skin specialist). Sometimes a biopsy (the removal of a tiny bit of the skin of the mouth where there's an ulcer) is needed to work out exactly what's going on – you will be referred to a hospital specialist for this.

Bowel disease Some diseases of the gut, such as ulcer-ative colitis and Crohn's disease (see the 'Diarrhoea' section, p. 50), can cause repeated attacks of mouth ulcers.

Treatment The ulcers themselves are treated in much the same way as aphthous ulcers (see above). For treatment of bowel disease, see the 'Diarrhoea' section (p. 50).

Blood disorder Serious blood diseases, like leukaemia, can very rarely show themselves through severe and persis-tent mouth ulcers, although there are usually lots of other symptoms too. The side-effects of some prescribed drugs (such as anti-thyroid and rheumatoid arthritis treatments) can cause blood problems, which also lead to mouth ulcers. If you're on one of these drugs, which is unlikely, you'll probably have been told to look out for this particular prob-lem and report it to your doctor.

Treatment See your GP urgently for a blood test.

Cancer Cancer of the lip, tongue, or mouth may start with a painless ulcer which slowly enlarges. This problem is very rare in the under 45s and may be linked with smoking and excess alcohol.

Treatment Any unexplained mouth ulcer which gets larger over weeks needs checking by your GP. If she's at all concerned, she'll refer you to a specialist for a biopsy (see above).

Multiple joint pains

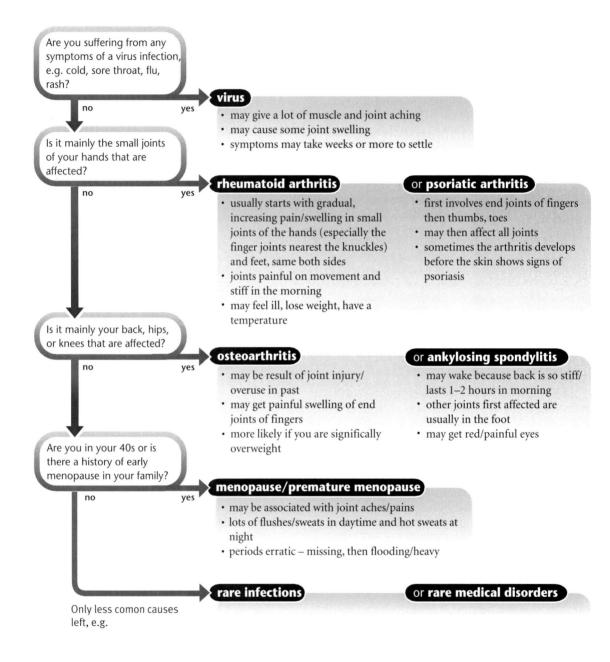

Are you suffering from any symptoms of a virus infection, e.g. cold, sore throat, flu, rash?

no / yes

virus
- may give a lot of muscle and joint aching
- may cause some joint swelling
- symptoms may take weeks or more to settle

Is it mainly the small joints of your hands that are affected?

no / yes

rheumatoid arthritis
- usually starts with gradual, increasing pain/swelling in small joints of the hands (especially the finger joints nearest the knuckles) and feet, same both sides
- joints painful on movement and stiff in the morning
- may feel ill, lose weight, have a temperature

or psoriatic arthritis
- first involves end joints of fingers then thumbs, toes
- may then affect all joints
- sometimes the arthritis develops before the skin shows signs of psoriasis

Is it mainly your back, hips, or knees that are affected?

no / yes

osteoarthritis
- may be result of joint injury/overuse in past
- may get painful swelling of end joints of fingers
- more likely if you are significantly overweight

or ankylosing spondylitis
- may wake because back is so stiff/lasts 1–2 hours in morning
- other joints first affected are usually in the foot
- may get red/painful eyes

Are you in your 40s or is there a history of early menopause in your family?

no / yes

menopause/premature menopause
- may be associated with joint aches/pains
- lots of flushes/sweats in daytime and hot sweats at night
- periods erratic – missing, then flooding/heavy

rare infections

or rare medical disorders

Only less comon causes left, e.g.

Virus A lot of viruses can result in joint aches, or even joint swellings, along with all the other symptoms they cause. Examples include flu, hepatitis, glandular fever, and German measles.

Treatment There is no magic cure for viruses – they just have to work their way out of the system. Joint pains can sometimes take a few weeks to settle down, and can be helped by anti-inflammatory drugs (such as ibuprofen – available from the chemist). You'll need to see your GP to check that the cause is a virus and for her to give you further advice depending on the particular germ you've been infected with.

Psoriatic arthritis A few people who suffer with psoriasis – a common skin condition causing a scaly rash – also get a particular type of arthritis. This usually affects the hands, although other joints can also cause trouble.

Treatment See your GP. If your arthritis isn't too bad, she may just treat you with anti-inflammatory drugs. But if they don't work, or your problem is severe, you'll be referred to the rheumatologist (joint specialist), who may need to use more powerful drugs to stop your joints getting too damaged.

Rheumatoid arthritis This type of arthritis usually starts between the ages of 30 and 50, initially affecting the hands, wrists, and feet. The exact cause is unknown.

Treatment If your GP thinks you may have this problem, she'll refer you to a rheumatologist. Rheumatoid arthritis can cause a lot of damage to your joints and to other parts of your body, so your specialist will give you advice about looking after your joints and will treat you with anti-inflammatory drugs or more powerful treatments to keep the arthritis at bay.

Menopause/premature menopause Some women find that the menopause causes or aggravates aches and pains in the joints. For further details, see the 'Flushing' section (p. 66).

Osteoarthritis This is 'wear and tear' type arthritis. It's common in older age groups – the majority of people aged over 50 have signs of osteoarthritis if their joints are X-rayed. But it's much less common in younger age groups. It can occur if you've made your joints suffer in the past (such as through a lot of heavy exercise like serious road running) or if you've had other joint problems (especially knee cartilage surgery) – in these situations, the knees and hips are the likeliest to have problems.

Treatment The main points in treating osteoarthritis can be found in the 'Osteoarthritis' part of the 'Knee pain' section (p.86).

Ankylosing spondylitis This uncommon form of arthritis affects people under the age of 30, causing low back pain and stiffness, pain in the joints of the rib cage and, sometimes, pain and swelling in other joints. The cause is unknown, though it sometimes runs in families.

Treatment This is another job for the rheumatologist. Apart from prescribing you various treatments, your specialist will advise you about keeping active and supple: it's very important to take regular exercise, such as swimming, and to improve your posture.

Rare infections Some pretty unusual infections can cause joint pains among their various other symptoms. These include gonorrhoea (a sexually transmitted germ which usually also results in a discharge from the vagina and/or burning on weeing), Lyme disease (caused by a tick bite), and brucellosis (a germ picked up from cattle, so a hazard to vets, abattoir workers, and so on).

Treatment See your GP – and tell her why you think you might have one of these rarities.

Other rare medical disorders There are a load of rare types of arthritis and small-print illnesses which can cause joint pains.

Treatment The chances are you haven't got any of them. If you're concerned, see your GP, who will run any necessary tests.

Nail problems

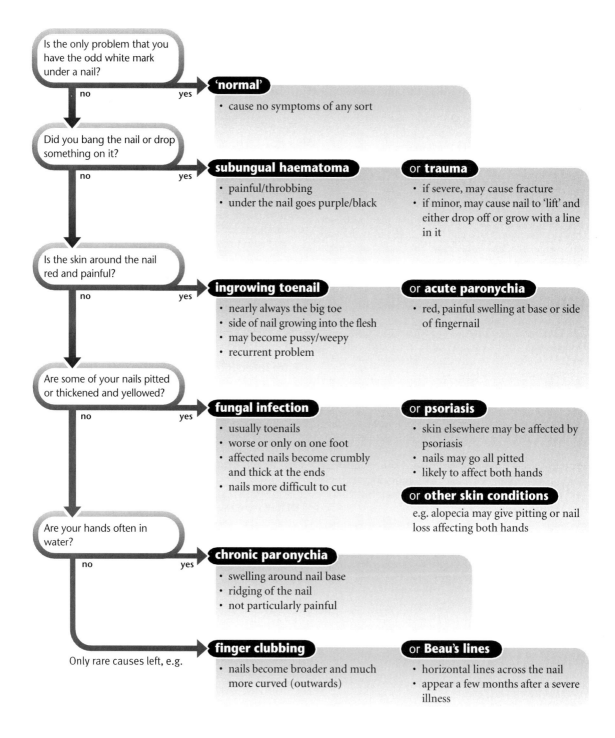

Is the only problem that you have the odd white mark under a nail?

'normal'
- cause no symptoms of any sort

no — yes

Did you bang the nail or drop something on it?

subungual haematoma
- painful/throbbing
- under the nail goes purple/black

or trauma
- if severe, may cause fracture
- if minor, may cause nail to 'lift' and either drop off or grow with a line in it

no — yes

Is the skin around the nail red and painful?

ingrowing toenail
- nearly always the big toe
- side of nail growing into the flesh
- may become pussy/weepy
- recurrent problem

or acute paronychia
- red, painful swelling at base or side of fingernail

no — yes

Are some of your nails pitted or thickened and yellowed?

fungal infection
- usually toenails
- worse or only on one foot
- affected nails become crumbly and thick at the ends
- nails more difficult to cut

or psoriasis
- skin elsewhere may be affected by psoriasis
- nails may go all pitted
- likely to affect both hands

or other skin conditions
e.g. alopecia may give pitting or nail loss affecting both hands

no — yes

Are your hands often in water?

chronic paronychia
- swelling around nail base
- ridging of the nail
- not particularly painful

no — yes

Only rare causes left, e.g.

finger clubbing
- nails become broader and much more curved (outwards)

or Beau's lines
- horizontal lines across the nail
- appear a few months after a severe illness

Normal marks The occasional white mark under one or more nails is quite normal. Contrary to popular belief, it doesn't suggest a lack of calcium, a vitamin deficiency, or any other problem, and so needs no treatment.

Subungual haematoma Blood under the nail. This happens after an injury – typically after jamming your finger in a door. Because the blood is under pressure, it's very painful.

Treatment If you can bear the pain, it's safe to leave it alone, as the blood will get reabsorbed after a few days. But if it's really throbbing and you're feeling brave, you can try making a hole in the nail. Simply heat up the tip of an unfolded paper clip or a pin until it's red hot. Then place the tip in the centre of your nail and grit your teeth. It will burn a hole through your nail and the blood, under pressure, will suddenly spurt out, giving you instant relief. The only pain you'll feel is when you finally get through the nail and touch the sensitive tissue underneath – this only lasts a second. Don't try this trick if you've really mangled your finger or thumb badly, though – if there's a broken bone, making a hole could introduce infection. Go to casualty instead.

Ingrowing toenail This almost always affects the big toe. The side of the nail grows into the flesh, which becomes swollen and sore. It can also get infected, making it hurt and swell more, and discharge pus.

Treatment Avoid narrow-toed shoes and cut the nail straight across rather than in a curve. An antiseptic cream may cure an early infection, but, if it's very mucky, sore, and swollen, you'll probably need antibiotics. But these only clear the infection, not the ingrowing nail itself. There are a couple of DIY treatments you can try. Cutting a tiny 'V' into the middle of the top of the nail makes it slightly more flexible – this relieves the pressure from the ingrowing edge. Alternatively, using the blunt end of a cocktail stick, wedge a plug of cotton wool soaked in disinfectant under the ingrowing part. Repeat this trick daily and you may be able to cure yourself, although, as the nail grows very slowly, it can take up to three months. If all else fails, your GP can arrange for you to have a minor operation to sort it out.

Acute paronychia An infection caused by a germ getting under the skin at the base of the nail.

Treatment If it's just started, see your GP for some antibiotics. But if it's gone on for a few days and the swelling is very tender and soft, it'll need lancing to let the pus out. This may be a GP or hospital job – give your doctor a ring and see what she says.

Trauma A minor injury can make the nail lift up as it grows out. Alternatively, it might develop a groove or ridge.

Treatment There's nothing you need to do about this. If the nail comes off, don't worry. It'll feel sore for a few days, but a new nail will grow.

Fungal infection A fungus can get into the nail and make it thicken and crumble.

Treatment These infections are difficult to clear, so if it's not bothering you, leave it alone. It might eventually go on its own, or you might just have to clip or file it down occasionally. If it's causing pain or you hate the way it looks, see your GP as there are anti-fungal tablets available which might cure the problem.

Psoriasis This is explained in the 'Rash' section (p. 126). Some people with psoriasis find it causes problems with their nails too, including small pits and thickening.

Treatment There is no effective treatment for this problem.

Other skin conditions Skin and nails are closely linked, so various skin problems, like hand eczema and alopecia areata (see 'Hair loss' section, p. 68), can also damage the nails.

Treatment Again, treatments don't really help at all.

Chronic paronychia If you frequently have your hands in water – maybe through your work or because he won't help with washing-up at home – the thin rim of skin at the base of the nail (the cuticle) may disappear. This allows a type of fungus to enter the skin, causing slight swelling around the nail base, and ridging of the nail itself. This is chronic paronychia.

Treatment The cure lies in keeping your hands out of water. If that's impossible, make sure you wear gloves with a cotton liner. An anti-fungal cream (such as clotrimazole, which is available from the chemist) applied to the swollen area may also help, though it may take weeks.

Rare problems Examples include Beau's lines and clubbing. Any severe illness can slow down nail growth. This results in horizontal lines (Beau's lines) appearing across all the nails (especially the fingernails). Usually, these only become noticeable a few months after the illness which has caused them. Various rare conditions (like lung or bowel disease) can affect the way the nails grow, resulting in nails which broaden and curve (in the direction of a claw). The fingertips may grow the same way too. This is known as 'clubbing'.

Treatment No treatment is needed for Beau's lines as they will grow out. If you've had clubbing since childbirth and it's in the family too, then it's a type handed down through the generations and is harmless. But if it's developed recently, see your GP. If she thinks there's a problem, she'll arrange any necessary tests.

Nipple discharge

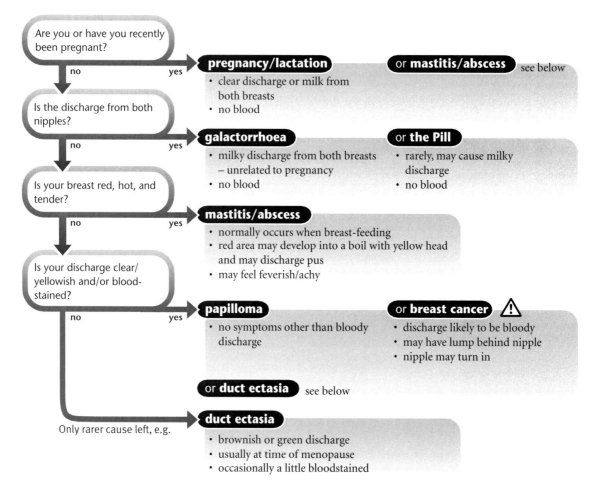

Are you or have you recently been pregnant?
no → (down)
yes → **pregnancy/lactation** • clear discharge or milk from both breasts • no blood — **or mastitis/abscess** see below

Is the discharge from both nipples?
no → (down)
yes → **galactorrhoea** • milky discharge from both breasts – unrelated to pregnancy • no blood — **or the Pill** • rarely, may cause milky discharge • no blood

Is your breast red, hot, and tender?
no → (down)
yes → **mastitis/abscess** • normally occurs when breast-feeding • red area may develop into a boil with yellow head and may discharge pus • may feel feverish/achy

Is your discharge clear/yellowish and/or blood-stained?
no → (down)
yes → **papilloma** • no symptoms other than bloody discharge — **or breast cancer** ⚠ • discharge likely to be bloody • may have lump behind nipple • nipple may turn in

or duct ectasia see below

Only rarer cause left, e.g. → **duct ectasia** • brownish or green discharge • usually at time of menopause • occasionally a little bloodstained

⚠ Regardless of the likely cause, any bloody discharge from the nipple should be checked by your GP.

Pregnancy/lactation The hormone changes in pregnancy which stimulate the breasts to enlarge can result in some discharge. Further hormone changes after childbirth – and, in the breast-feeding mother, the effect of the baby suckling – results in milk production ('lactation'). Even some time after breast-feeding has finished, it may still be possible to 'express' some milk from the breast. In fact, 'checking' to see if there's any milk left actually stimulates the breasts to produce more.

Treatment These situtations are quite normal and so need no treatment. If you're bottle-feeding your baby but are still troubled by leakage of milk from your nipples, then simply stop 'checking' your breasts and it'll soon clear up.

Galactorrhoea This means the production of a milky discharge from both breasts when it is 'not normal' – in other words, not just after childbirth. There are lots of different causes. The most common is stimulation of the breasts: this can cause milk production even some time after childbirth (see above). An active sex life with plenty of nipple stimulation can also lead to galactorrhoea. Other causes include the side-effects of medications (such as treatments used in some psychiatric problems), thyroid disorders and, occasionally, small brain tumours.

Treatment This problem needs checking by your GP and, possibly, blood tests or referral to a specialist.

Papilloma (or papillomas) This is a harmless warty growth inside one of the network of thin tubes which lie inside your breasts. You may have more than one papilloma, and they can bleed, causing a bloodstained discharge from the nipple.

Treatment A bloodstained discharge needs assessment by a specialist to check there isn't any serious problem with your breast – so see your GP as soon as possible.

Mastitis/abscess These problems are explained in the 'Breast pain' section (p. 40). They can result in some pus-like discharge from the nipple.

Treatment See the 'Breast pain' section (p. 40).

Duct ectasia As the breast ages, the thin tubes inside it can widen, clog, and become inflamed. This is known as 'duct ectasia' and is most common around the time of the menopause. The result is a brownish or green – and occasionally bloodstained – discharge.

Treatment This needs checking by your GP. She may be able to reassure you that all is well, or you may need to be assessed by a breast specialist.

The Pill The hormone changes caused by the Pill can very occasionally result in a milky discharge from both breasts.

Treatment The first step is to see your GP to check that this is the cause. Once the Pill has been confirmed as the problem, you have a choice – either carry on as before if the discharge doesn't bother you too much, or switch to another method of family planning.

Breast cancer It's unusual for cancer of the breast to show itself just as nipple discharge – especially if there is no blood in the discharge and you're under 50 years old. For more details, see the 'Breast lumps' section.

Treatment Check your symptoms with your GP. If she feels it needs further assessment to check for cancer, she'll refer you urgently to a breast specialist.

Noises in the ear

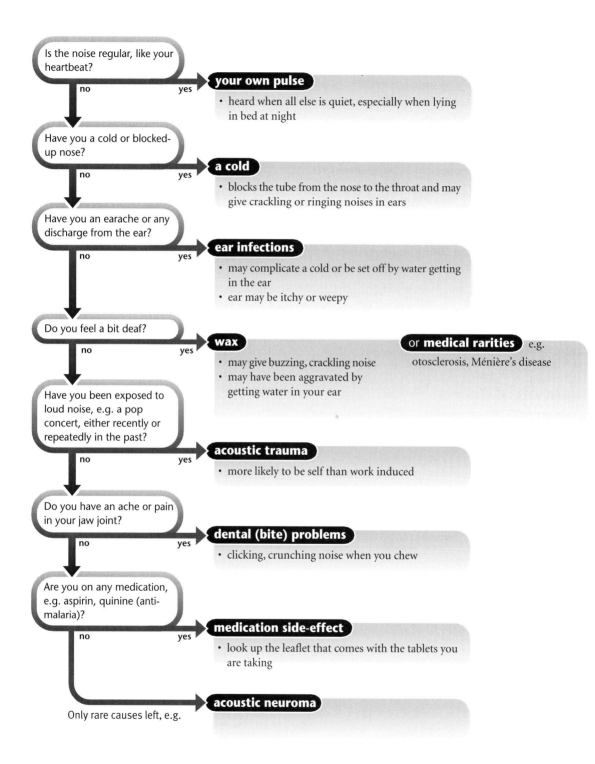

Is the noise regular, like your heartbeat?

no   yes

your own pulse
- heard when all else is quiet, especially when lying in bed at night

Have you a cold or blocked-up nose?

no   yes

a cold
- blocks the tube from the nose to the throat and may give crackling or ringing noises in ears

Have you an earache or any discharge from the ear?

no   yes

ear infections
- may complicate a cold or be set off by water getting in the ear
- ear may be itchy or weepy

Do you feel a bit deaf?

no   yes

wax
- may give buzzing, crackling noise
- may have been aggravated by getting water in your ear

or medical rarities e.g. otosclerosis, Ménière's disease

Have you been exposed to loud noise, e.g. a pop concert, either recently or repeatedly in the past?

no   yes

acoustic trauma
- more likely to be self than work induced

Do you have an ache or pain in your jaw joint?

no   yes

dental (bite) problems
- clicking, crunching noise when you chew

Are you on any medication, e.g. aspirin, quinine (anti-malaria)?

no   yes

medication side-effect
- look up the leaflet that comes with the tablets you are taking

acoustic neuroma

Only rare causes left, e.g.

Noises in the ear

Your own pulse Most of the time, you won't be aware of this – but if everything is quiet (usually at night), you may hear the pulse in your ear. This is most likely to happen if your pulse is harder or faster than usual, such as if you're anxious or have a fever.

Treatment This is normal and so needs no treatment. Turning over on to the other side may get rid of it if it's bothering you when you're lying in bed.

A cold Caused by a virus and inflames the ear, nose, and throat. Catarrh tends to block the inner tubes causing pressure changes in your ears, making them feel as though they want to 'pop'. Pressure on the eardrums produces a sensation of ringing in the ears (tinnitus).

Treatment There is no magic cure for a cold, so there's no point seeing your GP. The symptoms will disappear after a few days. The stuffed-up feeling and noises in the ears may be helped by steam inhalations – put a towel over your head, then put your head over a bowl of hot water and breathe in the steam.

Ear wax This is explained in the section on 'Deafness' (p. 48). Wax can press on the eardrum, causing tinnitus.

Treatment See the section on 'Deafness' (p. 48).

Ear infections There are different types of infections which can affect the ear. Some just cause problems with the ear canal, others go deeper and affect the eardrum and beyond. Some are 'one-offs', others keep coming back, and others stay there constantly until dealt with by your GP or a specialist. They can all cause an ear discharge and this, together with possible damage to the drum and other parts of the ear, can lead to tinnitus.

Treatment A GP job to sort out the type of infection and prescribe you the right treatment – probably either drops or antibiotics. You might have to see an Ear, Nose, and Throat ('ENT') specialist if the infection is difficult to shift or causing a lot of problems. For the future, you can keep problems to a minimum by avoiding cotton buds and keeping water out of your ears – so use ear plugs or a wedge of cotton wool dipped in vaseline when you're swimming or washing your hair.

Acoustic trauma This means damage caused by loud noises. It's normal to feel ringing in the ears after a sudden loud noise, such as an explosion – this usually goes away quickly. Repeated exposure to noise, such as working in a noisy environment without ear protection, or too much clubbing, can damage the ear, resulting in long-term tinnitus and deafness.

Treatment It's important to protect the ears from further problems by wearing ear protection at work and cutting down on raucous music through earphones. Unfortunately, tinnitus of this sort cannot be cured. If it's causing you real problems, it's worth talking to your GP. Treatments that can help include masking devices (aids which produce a 'white noise', blocking out the tinnitus), psychological help (to train you how to relax and ignore the noise), and antidepressants (if the symptom is really getting you down).

Dental problems Dental trouble, especially if it puts the 'bite' of your upper and lower teeth out of line, can inflame the jaw joint (the temporomandibular joint). As a result, you'll notice clicking and crunching sounds, particularly when you chew.

Treatment Bite the bullet and see your dentist.

Medication side-effect Over-the-counter treatments such as aspirin and ibuprofen, and prescribed drugs like quinine (used for cramps and prevention of malaria for travellers abroad), can produce tinnitus as a side-effect – especially if you take more than the recommended dose.

Treatment Stop the offending drug. If you've accidentally or deliberately exceeded the stated dose, get urgent medical help by going straight to casualty.

Medical rarities There are some uncommon illnesses which can cause ringing in the ears. These include Ménière's disease (raised pressure of the fluid deep in the ears), otosclerosis (seizing up of the tiny bones in the ear), and acoustic neuroma (a growth on the nerve leading away from the ear).

Treatment See your GP. If she's concerned, she'll send you to an ENT specialist for tests and treatment.

Odd behaviour

NB The problem here is that you may not think your behaviour is odd at all because, in some of the more serious conditions, you lose touch with reality. So hand the book over to your nearest and dearest, and let them sort you out.

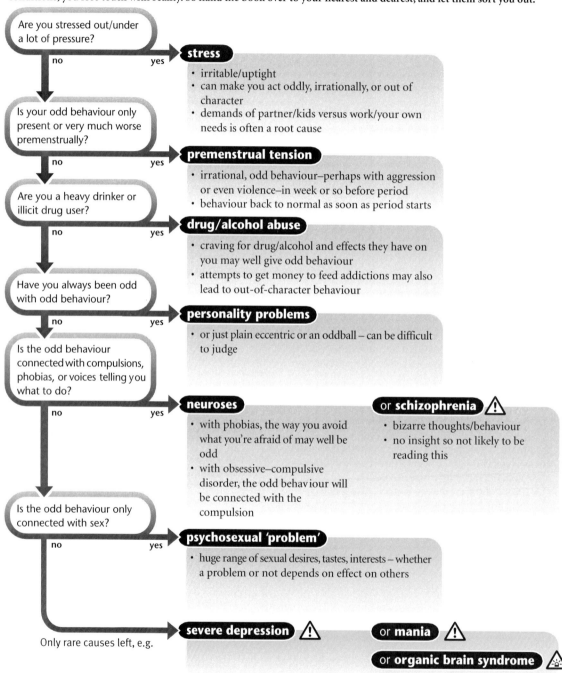

Are you stressed out/under a lot of pressure?

no / yes

stress
- irritable/uptight
- can make you act oddly, irrationally, or out of character
- demands of partner/kids versus work/your own needs is often a root cause

Is your odd behaviour only present or very much worse premenstrually?

no / yes

premenstrual tension
- irrational, odd behaviour–perhaps with aggression or even violence–in week or so before period
- behaviour back to normal as soon as period starts

Are you a heavy drinker or illicit drug user?

no / yes

drug/alcohol abuse
- craving for drug/alcohol and effects they have on you may well give odd behaviour
- attempts to get money to feed addictions may also lead to out-of-character behaviour

Have you always been odd with odd behaviour?

no / yes

personality problems
- or just plain eccentric or an oddball – can be difficult to judge

Is the odd behaviour connected with compulsions, phobias, or voices telling you what to do?

no / yes

neuroses
- with phobias, the way you avoid what you're afraid of may well be odd
- with obsessive–compulsive disorder, the odd behaviour will be connected with the compulsion

or schizophrenia ⚠
- bizarre thoughts/behaviour
- no insight so not likely to be reading this

Is the odd behaviour only connected with sex?

no / yes

psychosexual 'problem'
- huge range of sexual desires, tastes, interests – whether a problem or not depends on effect on others

Only rare causes left, e.g.

severe depression ⚠   **or mania** ⚠

or organic brain syndrome ⚠

⚠ If you are a diabetic, treat odd behaviour as hypoglycaemia until proved otherwise.

Stress Being under pressure all the time – typically because of work, relationship, or money worries – will make you feel constantly uptight. The result is usually a short fuse: it won't take much to make you explode, so you may experience outbursts of anger or you may even get violent. Alternatively, you might get depressed and weepy.

Treatment Look at the 'Feeling tense' (p. 64) or 'Feeling down' (p. 62) section, depending on whether you're feeling uptight or depressed.

Drug and alcohol abuse Mind-expanding drugs will obviously alter your behaviour. Alcohol does the same. Suddenly stopping after long-term use can cause a 'withdrawal syndrome', with cravings, physical symptoms, and odd behaviour. Also, in the long run, being hooked on drugs or booze can change your personality, because you'll lead a chaotic lifestyle – for example, you may become short tempered, devious, and suspicious of other people.

Treatment Cut down on the drugs and booze – and preferably stop them altogether. If you think you need help, see your GP or contact the local drug or alcohol unit.

Personality problems It's a matter of opinion when a personality crosses the line from being normal to abnormal. But psychiatrists do recognize certain types of personality which, when extreme, can cause problems, either to the individual or to those around her. These include the psychopath (aggressive, often in trouble with the law, antisocial) and the paranoid (oversensitive and suspicious), although there are many others. The cause of these exaggerated personalities is probably a mixture of family traits and a disturbed childhood.

Treatment Personalities can't be changed, so there's no 'cure', but psychologists and psychiatrists can sometimes help people to alter their behaviour – speak to your GP.

Neuroses These are a variety of psychiatric problems which all result in anxiety. They include, among others, phobias and panic attacks. They are explained in more detail, and their treatments discussed, in the 'Feeling tense' section (p. 64).

Premenstrual tension Odd behaviour, such as acting impulsively or having an unreasonably short fuse, may be caused by the feelings of tension which occur in women who suffer severely from premenstrual syndrome.

Treatment This is discussed in the 'Feeling tense' section (p. 64).

Schizophrenia This is a serious psychiatric problem causing a pattern of odd symptoms and behaviour (see flow chart). It usually starts in your early 20s and its cause is unknown, although it may result from chemical imbalances in the brain.

Treatment This needs the help of your GP, who, in turn, will probably call in a psychiatrist. You may not realize you're ill; you might even need to be 'forced' to go into hospital under the Mental Health Act (a law which enables doctors to insist that you have treatment even when you don't want it). Medication is usually in the form of tablets and injections. Unfortunately, the problem tends to come back, so you'll need ongoing help and monitoring from your GP, psychiatrist, or a mental health nurse.

Depression This is explained, and its treatment outlined, in the 'Feeling down' section (p. 62). Serious depression can, very occasionally, make you lose touch with reality, develop bizarre, negative thoughts, and behave oddly.

Psychosexual problem There is an astonishing range of odd sexual behaviour (ranging from fetishism to bondage). What is regarded as 'abnormal' depends on your partner, society, and the law.

Treatment If your psychosexual problem is causing you, or others, problems, speak to your GP. She will probably refer you to a psychosexual counsellor (a 'sexpert') or a psychiatrist.

Mania This is another serious psychiatric problem in which you totally lose touch with reality. It tends to keep coming back and may alternate with attacks of depression. The cause is unknown.

Treatment Much the same as for schizophrenia (see above). Medication can also be used to try to prevent attacks.

Organic brain syndrome This is any physical illness which clouds how the brain works. There are many of causes. Some are sudden (e.g. a head injury or meningitis) and others are gradual (e.g. a brain tumour or Creutzfeldt-Jakob disease [CJD]). A few medications can, rarely, have the same effect (e.g. steroids and some blood pressure pills). In diabetics on treatment, a common cause is hypoglycaemia (a low blood sugar) caused, for example, by a missed meal or excess exercise.

Treatment These situations obviously require medical attention – urgently in the case of problems with a sudden onset. If you're a diabetic and you think you're having a 'hypo', get some sugar down you asap.

Pain in the ankle, foot, or toe

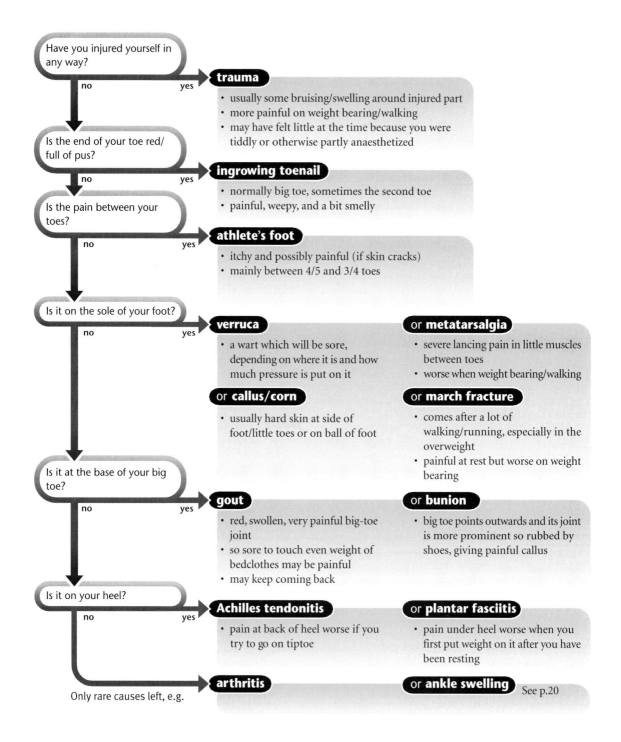

Have you injured yourself in any way?

no / yes

trauma
- usually some bruising/swelling around injured part
- more painful on weight bearing/walking
- may have felt little at the time because you were tiddly or otherwise partly anaesthetized

Is the end of your toe red/full of pus?

no / yes

ingrowing toenail
- normally big toe, sometimes the second toe
- painful, weepy, and a bit smelly

Is the pain between your toes?

no / yes

athlete's foot
- itchy and possibly painful (if skin cracks)
- mainly between 4/5 and 3/4 toes

Is it on the sole of your foot?

no / yes

verruca
- a wart which will be sore, depending on where it is and how much pressure is put on it

or callus/corn
- usually hard skin at side of foot/little toes or on ball of foot

or metatarsalgia
- severe lancing pain in little muscles between toes
- worse when weight bearing/walking

or march fracture
- comes after a lot of walking/running, especially in the overweight
- painful at rest but worse on weight bearing

Is it at the base of your big toe?

no / yes

gout
- red, swollen, very painful big-toe joint
- so sore to touch even weight of bedclothes may be painful
- may keep coming back

or bunion
- big toe points outwards and its joint is more prominent so rubbed by shoes, giving painful callus

Is it on your heel?

no / yes

Achilles tendonitis
- pain at back of heel worse if you try to go on tiptoe

or plantar fasciitis
- pain under heel worse when you first put weight on it after you have been resting

Only rare causes left, e.g.

arthritis

or ankle swelling See p.20

Trauma For ankle injuries, see the 'Ankle swelling' section (p. 20). Twisting your ankle can cause other injuries, such as a bit of bone being pulled off the outer edge of your foot.

Treatment If you may have broken a bone – a severe injury, a lot of bruising, and swelling or you can't bear weight – you need to go to casualty. Otherwise, if it's really sore, use ice-packs and painkillers and rest the injured part for a day or two.

Athlete's foot This is an infection between the webs of the toes caused by a fungus. It's usually itchy, but it can be sore if it makes the skin crack.

Treatment Keep your feet dry and use an anti-fungal cream from the chemist.

Ingrowing toenail A nail which curves into the skin, making it swollen and sore. It can get infected, in which case it goes red, gets more painful, and leaks pus.

Treatment Avoid narrow-toed shoes and cut the nail straight across rather than in a curve. Try a couple of DIY tricks: wedge a plug of antiseptic-soaked cotton wool under the ingrowing edge each day – this 'persuades' the nail to grow out of the skin, but takes weeks or even months to work. Or you can cut a small 'V' in the middle of the front edge of the nail, as this relieves the pressure on the sides. If it gets infected, you'll need antibiotics from your GP – and if you get problems for months without any signs of improvement, talk to her about a small operation to sort it out.

Verruca This is a wart growing into the sole of the foot.

Treatment It's best to leave it alone as it'll go on its own eventually. If it's a nuisance, soak the foot each evening to soften the skin, then rub the verruca with a pumice stone – keep this up for a few weeks and you may succeed in filing it down to nothing.

Callus/corn This is hard skin caused by friction. It may develop on the sole of the foot or where one toe rubs against another.

Treatment As for a verruca (see above).

Bunion If your big toe starts to point in towards your other toes, its base sticks out and gets rubbed by your shoes. This makes the base of the toe inflamed.

Treatment If it's a problem, try pads to relieve the pressure or strapping to straighten the toe (both available from the chemist). If you're desperate, surgery can help.

Achilles tendonitis The Achilles tendon is the tough, thick cord connecting your calf to your heel. 'Tendonitis' is inflammation of the tendon – usually the result of overdoing exercise or the heel tab of your trainer rubbing on it.

Treatment Rest for a few weeks then gradually start exercising again, avoiding trainers with high heel tabs. Anti-inflammatory drugs (available over the counter) may help.

Metatarsalgia This is pain in the ball of the foot. It has a number of causes, including new shoes, too much running, and a trapped nerve.

Treatment Padding under the ball of the foot and anti-inflammatory drugs may help. If the problem persists, see your GP for further advice and treatment.

Plantar fasciitis An inflammation of the sole of the foot (mainly the heel area). Again, this can be caused by new shoes or by doing unusual amounts of walking or running.

Treatment A heel pad and anti-inflammatories may help. Otherwise, you'll probably need a cortisone injection, so see your GP.

Ankle swelling Anything which makes your ankle (or ankles) swell may cause discomfort too. For further details, see 'Ankle swelling' section (p. 20).

March fracture A stress fracture of a bone in the foot – usually caused by excess running on hard surfaces.

Treatment This needs about six weeks' rest, then a gradual return to exercise – preferably with better shoes and on a softer surface.

Gout In your blood there is a chemical called 'uric acid'. In some people, the level of this chemical is high enough for them to develop uric acid crystals, which get stuck in joints (especially the big-toe joint), causing severe inflammation. It may run in families and it's aggravated by being overweight or drinking too much alcohol – but it's very unusual in women before the menopause.

Treatment If it's your first attack, you're bound to see your doctor as it's so painful. Rest the toe, and use ice-packs and the anti-inflammatory drug your GP will prescribe. Keep some handy in case you get further attacks. To cut the chances of further problems, shed any excess pounds and don't overdo the alcohol. If you do keep getting attacks, see your GP, as she may prescribe you treatment to try to prevent the problem.

Arthritis Various types of arthritis can affect the ankles (see the 'Ankle swelling' (p. 20) and 'Multiple joint pains' (p. 100) sections). Osteoarthritis (wear and tear) can affect the big toe.

Treatment For ankle problems, see the sections mentioned above. Big-toe arthritis is usually helped by painkillers and padding.

Pain in the bottom

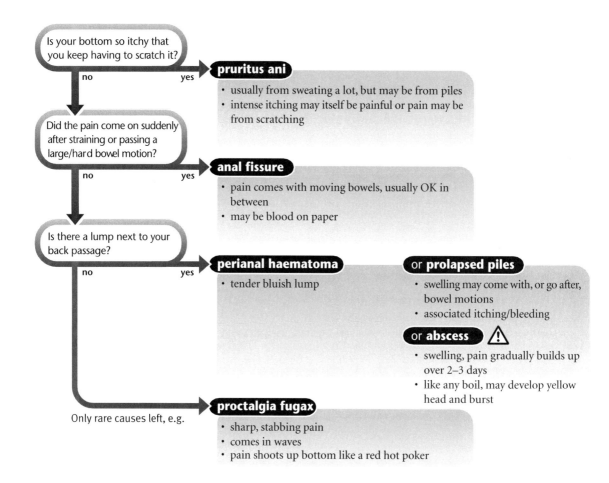

Is your bottom so itchy that you keep having to scratch it?

no / yes

pruritus ani
- usually from sweating a lot, but may be from piles
- intense itching may itself be painful or pain may be from scratching

Did the pain come on suddenly after straining or passing a large/hard bowel motion?

no / yes

anal fissure
- pain comes with moving bowels, usually OK in between
- may be blood on paper

Is there a lump next to your back passage?

no / yes

perianal haematoma
- tender bluish lump

or prolapsed piles
- swelling may come with, or go after, bowel motions
- associated itching/bleeding

or abscess ⚠
- swelling, pain gradually builds up over 2–3 days
- like any boil, may develop yellow head and burst

Only rare causes left, e.g.

proctalgia fugax
- sharp, stabbing pain
- comes in waves
- pain shoots up bottom like a red hot poker

Remember: ⚠ means see your GP sharpish; ⚠ means an urgent hospital job

Pruritus ani This is the medical term for itching around the tail-end. It can get very sore, especially if you scratch it a lot. There are lots of different things that can cause it in the first place, such as sweating and eczema, but it's the scratching which keeps it going by inflaming the sensitive skin.

Treatment There are two key steps to sorting this out. First, keep the area clean and dry – the easiest way is to use wet-wipes to clean thoroughly each time you open your bowels. Second, stop scratching – it won't have a chance to heal up if you're tearing the skin to pieces. You can also try small amounts of hydrocortisone 1% cream from the chemist twice a day, as this will ease the itching. If all else fails, discuss the problem with your doc, as you may need a 'prescription-only' cream, or some other treatment, to sort it out.

Perianal haematoma A burst blood vessel next to the back passage. The blood leaks into, and stretches, the skin, giving a tender, bluish, cherry-sized lump (technically, a 'haematoma'). It's usually caused by straining when you're constipated, or by a bout of diarrhoea.

Treatment It will go away on its own after five days or so. You'll be left with a tiny soft lump – a 'skin tag' – which is harmless and so can be ignored. Because the haematoma hurts, it's tempting to avoid opening your bowels regularly – but you must, otherwise you'll get constipated, and any straining runs the risk of developing another one straight away. If the pain is agonizing, consider going to casualty, as it's possible to have the lump cut open so that the blood inside can be shelled out, relieving the pressure. On the other hand, you might just want to grit your teeth for a few days. It's certainly worth increasing your fibre intake for the future, to cut down the chance of further problems.

Anal fissure A small tear in the back passage. The causes are the same as for a perianal haematoma (see above).

Treatment This, too, will usually sort itself out, though it may take a week or two. Again, it's important not to let the pain get you constipated – straining will open up the split again. If possible, have a quick dunk in a bath each time you've opened your bowels, as this will ease the pain and help keep the area clean. You can also try lignocaine gel or ointment (an anaesthetic) from the chemist – rub it into the sore area about half an hour before, and shortly after, going to the toilet. Very occasionally, the fissure won't heal. So if it's going on for weeks without improving, see your GP. You may need to be referred to a specialist for a small operation.

Prolapsed piles Piles are simply varicose veins (swollen blood vessels) in the back passage (see 'Lumps in the back passage' section, p. 96). They aren't usually painful, but if they drop down and poke out of your bottom – in other words, prolapse – they can get sore.

Treatment If they pop back in after you've been to the toilet, they're unlikely to cause you too many problems. Simply avoid getting too constipated (as above). If they stay out all the time, they're more likely to cause pain and bleeding. Any of the heaps of creams available from the chemist will help the soreness, but they're likely to need other treatment – possibly a small operation – so see your GP. Very occasionally, prolapsed piles which stay out can become 'strangulated' – throttled by the muscle of your back passage. This causes severe pain and swelling: next stop, casualty.

Abscess A skin infection which can develop into a large, hot, painful lump.

Treatment An abscess needs, at best, a course of antibiotics and, at worst, a trip to the hospital for lancing. So see your doctor – urgently if the lump is large, very painful, and you feel unwell and feverish.

Proctalgia fugax A severe pain in the back passage. The bad news is that no one knows what causes it. The good news is that it's harmless.

Treatment A really tough one. There is no cure and no consistently effective treatment. Some find hot baths useful, others use ice-packs, and some find massage in or around the back passage stops an attack. Otherwise it's a case of either dosing yourself up with a strong painkiller or seeing if your GP might try you on a prescribed treatment – some doctors have found that an ointment usually used to treat angina seems to help proctalgia when applied to the tail-end (just don't ask how they discovered this).

Painful periods

N.B. If you do not normally have painful periods but get what you think is 'severe period pain', it may be pain from something else, like appendicitis, which is nothing to do with your period – see 'Abdominal pain – one-off' (p.8) or 'Lower abdominal pain – one-off' (p.92) sections.

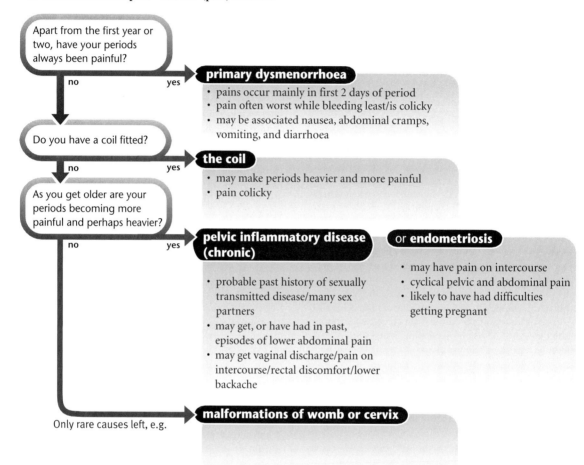

Apart from the first year or two, have your periods always been painful?

no   yes

primary dysmenorrhoea
- pains occur mainly in first 2 days of period
- pain often worst while bleeding least/is colicky
- may be associated nausea, abdominal cramps, vomiting, and diarrhoea

Do you have a coil fitted?

no   yes

the coil
- may make periods heavier and more painful
- pain colicky

As you get older are your periods becoming more painful and perhaps heavier?

no   yes

pelvic inflammatory disease (chronic)
- probable past history of sexually transmitted disease/many sex partners
- may get, or have had in past, episodes of lower abdominal pain
- may get vaginal discharge/pain on intercourse/rectal discomfort/lower backache

or endometriosis
- may have pain on intercourse
- cyclical pelvic and abdominal pain
- likely to have had difficulties getting pregnant

Only rare causes left, e.g.

malformations of womb or cervix

Primary dysmenorrhoea This is the medical term for period pains not caused by any specific disease – in other words, 'normal' period pains. How severe they are obviously varies from woman to woman and, though 'normal', they can sometimes be incapacitating. The pain is caused by the womb contracting during the period.

Treatment This depends on how much the problem bothers you – you might just want reassurance that the symptoms aren't a sign of some gynaecological disease. If in doubt, see your GP. Mild pains may not need any treatment at all other than the occasional painkiller. For more severe problems, there is plenty of help available. The anti-inflammatory drug ibuprofen (available over the counter), taken at the time of your period, is often very effective at relieving pain. If this doesn't help, see your GP – she may try a different anti-inflammatory drug. Alternatively, if you also need contraception, she may suggest you go on the Pill as this is usually very effective.

Chronic pelvic inflammatory disease This is explained, and the treatment outlined, in the 'Lower abdominal pain – recurrent' section (p. 94).

Endometriosis This explained, and the treatment outlined, in the 'Lower abdominal pain – recurrent' section (p. 94).

Intrauterine contraceptive device ('the coil') The coil usually consists of a small piece of plastic encased in some copper. It is inserted through the cervix (neck of the womb) into the womb and needs replacing every five years or so. It is a very effective contraceptive but it may cause painful (and heavier) periods – young women who have had no previous pregnancies are particularly likely to find it makes their periods more painful.

Treatment It's worth getting your GP to check your coil, as painful periods can be a sign that it's not quite in the correct position. If all is well and you've only recently had the coil fitted, it's worth persevering – the problem often settles down after a few months. You can also try anti-inflammatory treatment such as ibuprofen (see above). But if you're getting nowhere and the symptoms are a real nuisance, you may need to have the coil removed and use a different form of family planning.

Other rare causes Unusual causes, such as polyps of the womb and narrowing of the neck of the womb, can very occasionally cause painful periods.

Treatment A problem like this is unlikely to be the cause of your symptoms. If it could be, your GP is likely to refer you to a gynaecologist.

Palpitations

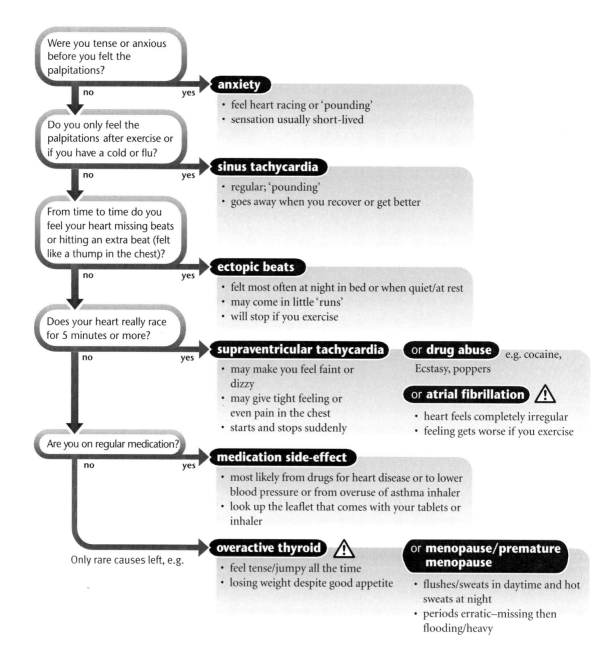

Anxiety People suffering from anxiety become more aware of their heartbeat and sometimes think their heart is racing or pounding even when it is beating perfectly normally. If you feel very tense, it's quite normal for the heart to beat faster than usual – most people notice this when they're in a situation which is making them nervous, such as making a speech. These sensations are often described as 'palpitations'.

Treatment It's important to realize that these sensations are harmless – otherwise, you might worry that there is something wrong with your heart, which will raise the anxiety levels even higher, causing more palpitations. If you're feeling tense most of the time, try to get to the root of the problem by sorting out the stressful areas of your life. Increasing your physical exercise, using relaxation techniques, and cutting down your caffeine intake (e.g. tea, coffee, and cola) may help. If the problem is causing you real difficulties and only happens in certain, predictable situations – such as when you have to give a presentation at work – it's worth seeing your GP. She might be able to advise about other relaxation techniques, or send you to see someone to help manage your anxiety. Or, if you're desperate, she might prescribe you something which will ease the palpitations and which you'll probably only have to take occasionally – whenever you're in the situation which brings on the palpitations.

Sinus tachycardia This is a heart which is beating appropriately fast. The normal rate is between 60 and 100 beats per minute. In sinus tachycardia, the rate is usually between 100 and 140 beats per minute. It happens, for example, after exercise or during a fever. The body needs more oxygen, so the heart pumps the blood around faster – hence the raised rate.

Treatment This is a normal response of the heart and so, in itself, does not require any treatment at all.

Ectopic beats The heart normally beats regularly, but it's quite normal for it to miss beats or throw in a few 'extra' beats occasionally. These odd irregular beats are not a sign of heart disease and are more noticeable, and sometimes more frequent, when you are stressed – they are the cause of the well-known 'butterflies in the stomach' sensation.

Treatment Usually, no specific treatment is needed – especially once you realize they're totally harmless. If they bother you, try the relaxation techniques outlined above. It's also worth cutting down on caffeine, alcohol, and smoking, all of which may aggravate the problem.

Supraventricular tachycardia The heart contains its own natural pacemaker which keeps it beating at the usual rates. Occasionally, a temporary 'short circuit' occurs, resulting in the heart beating much faster than normal. As for most of the other causes of palpitations, it's not usually caused by any disease of the heart.

Treatment Most attacks stop within half an hour or so. If it lasts longer or makes you feel very unwell, then get someone to take you to hospital for treatment to slow the rate back to normal. Some people who get repeated attacks discover tricks which can stop an attack – these include sticking your fingers down your throat to make yourself gag, or quickly swallowing something very cold (such as a large lump of ice cream). There are tablets which can be taken to prevent attacks so if you get repeated problems, see your GP, who will arrange any necessary tests and may start you on treatment.

Drug abuse Certain illicit drugs, such as cocaine, Ecstasy, poppers (amyl nitrite), and amphetamines, can make the heart race.

Treatment Although unpleasant, your racing pulse itself shouldn't cause you any problems – unless you already have heart trouble, which, in the under 45s, is unlikely. Obviously, the only way to cure these types of palpitation is to avoid the offending drug.

Medication side-effect A side-effect of some prescribed treatments is a speeding up of the heart rate. The most likely culprit is an asthma inhaler (such as salbutamol or terbutaline) – especially if it is used more often than recommended. Some blood pressure tablets can also cause palpitations.

Treatment If you feel that a prescribed medication you are taking might be causing palpitations, discuss the situation with your GP.

Overactive thyroid This is explained, and its treatment outlined, in the 'Excess sweating' section (p. 58).

Menopause/premature menopause The hormone changes of the menopause can cause, among other symptoms, palpitations – for further details, see the 'Flushing' section.

Atrial fibrillation This involves the heart beating rapidly and irregularly. It is very rare in the under 45s, in whom excess alcohol is the likeliest cause.

Treatment This requires medication from your GP – and a reduction in alcohol intake if that is the cause.

Pins and needles and numbness

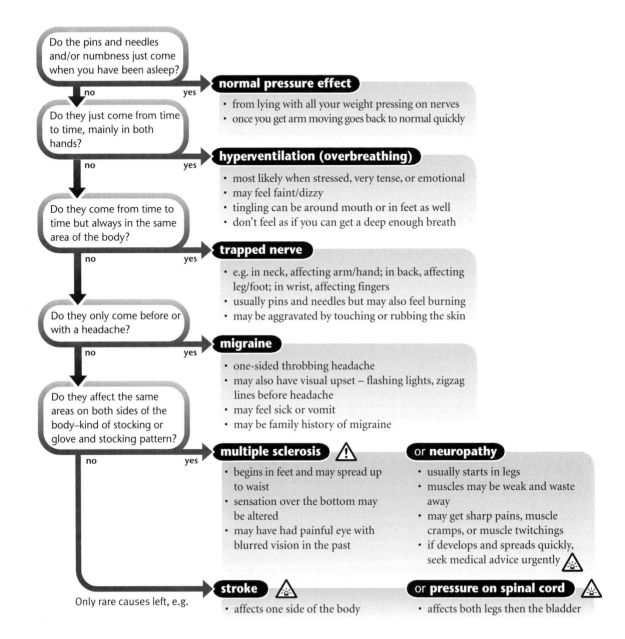

Do the pins and needles and/or numbness just come when you have been asleep? — no / yes

normal pressure effect
- from lying with all your weight pressing on nerves
- once you get arm moving goes back to normal quickly

Do they just come from time to time, mainly in both hands? — no / yes

hyperventilation (overbreathing)
- most likely when stressed, very tense, or emotional
- may feel faint/dizzy
- tingling can be around mouth or in feet as well
- don't feel as if you can get a deep enough breath

Do they come from time to time but always in the same area of the body? — no / yes

trapped nerve
- e.g. in neck, affecting arm/hand; in back, affecting leg/foot; in wrist, affecting fingers
- usually pins and needles but may also feel burning
- may be aggravated by touching or rubbing the skin

Do they only come before or with a headache? — no / yes

migraine
- one-sided throbbing headache
- may also have visual upset – flashing lights, zigzag lines before headache
- may feel sick or vomit
- may be family history of migraine

Do they affect the same areas on both sides of the body–kind of stocking or glove and stocking pattern? — no / yes

multiple sclerosis
- begins in feet and may spread up to waist
- sensation over the bottom may be altered
- may have had painful eye with blurred vision in the past

or neuropathy
- usually starts in legs
- muscles may be weak and waste away
- may get sharp pains, muscle cramps, or muscle twitchings
- if develops and spreads quickly, seek medical advice urgently

Only rare causes left, e.g.

stroke
- affects one side of the body

or pressure on spinal cord
- affects both legs then the bladder

⚠ If you are on the Pill and for the first time ever develop a migraine headache with pins and needles/numbness, then stop the Pill and arrange an appointment with your doctor for as soon as possible.

Normal pressure effect Most people have experienced waking in the night or first thing in the morning with a numb, 'dead', or tingly hand or arm, which comes back to normal after a minute or two. This is caused by the weight of your body temporarily trapping a nerve or affecting the circulation.

Treatment This is normal, harmless, and needs no treatment.

Hyperventilation This means breathing too fast and too deep and is usually part of a panic attack (see the 'Shortness of breath' section, p. 132). You end up getting too much oxygen into your system, which affects your nerves, causing pins and needles.

Treatment The way to cure an attack is simply to breathe in and out of a brown paper bag. This way, you breathe back in your own air, which doesn't have so much oxygen in it as fresh air, so you don't overdose on oxygen. Also try to breathe slowly and not too deeply. It's very important that people around you understand that these attacks are harmless – if they panic, it'll make you worse. Getting panic attacks is usually brought on by stress – see the 'Shortness of breath' section (p. 132) for further advice on how to handle the problem.

Trapped nerve The nerves which supply feeling to your skin start from the spinal cord and then travel through various channels and tunnels in muscles and bones to reach their final destination. They can get pressed on (or 'trapped') at any point in their journey. The obvious example is when you hurt your 'funny bone' – a nerve passes through your elbow where you tend to knock it, so it's momentarily trapped, causing pins and needles in your hand. This goes away after a few seconds, but some nerves can be trapped for days or even weeks. Examples include nerves in the neck (causing problems in the arm and hand), and a large nerve in the back (trapped when you slip a disc – 'sciatica' – causing numbness in your leg or foot). A nerve in the wrist can also get trapped – especially if you've put on weight or are pregnant – causing pins and needles or pain in the hand ('carpal tunnel syndrome').

Treatment A trapped nerve will usually sort itself out within a week or so. If it's painful or showing no signs of going, an anti-inflammatory drug like ibuprofen (available from the chemist) sometimes helps. But if it goes on for weeks without showing signs of improvement, gets worse, or causes weakness as well as numbness, see your GP – this will need checking out further and, if it is a trapped nerve, may need the help of a specialist to free it. For further information on sciatica, see 'Back pain' (p. 00). Carpal tunnel syndrome may be helped by dieting if you're overweight – and if caused by pregnancy, will go once you've had the baby. Otherwise, it can be helped by tablets, an injection, or even surgery, so see your GP if it's a real nuisance.

Migraine This is explained in the 'Headache' section (p. 70). Before the blood vessels to the brain widen, causing the migraine, they sometimes narrow. This starves the brain of oxygen for a short while, with the result that you might feel numbness somewhere on one side of your body just before, or with, the headache.

Treatment See the 'Migraine' part of the 'Headache' section (p. 70).

Multiple sclerosis This is caused by the insulation around your nerves (which is just like the insulation around electrical wiring) dying off. Lots of different nerves can be affected, though not all at the same time, causing a variety of symptoms – including pins and needles or numbness – which usually come and go. What actually causes multiple sclerosis in the first place is still unknown.

Treatment If you think you have multiple sclerosis, you need to see your GP – but you're much more likely to have one of the other causes described above. If your GP is concerned, she'll refer you to a neurologist (nerve specialist).

Neuropathy Lots of different medical problems can damage the nerves supplying the sensation to your skin, causing numbness or pins and needles. These include diabetes, excess alcohol, vitamin deficiencies, and some medications. Rarely, it may develop suddenly, perhaps a week or two after an infection (like a cold or tummy bug) and spread up your arms and legs and over the body. This is called Guillain–Barré syndrome.

Treatment See your GP. If she thinks you have a neuropathy, she'll run some blood tests to check it out, and will treat you according to what these tests show. If you think you might be developing Guillain–Barré syndrome, seek medical help urgently – this problem needs hospital treatment.

Other medical problems Some rare problems can cause pins and needles and numbness. These include strokes (which affect one half of the body, usually without a headache, for more than 24 hours) and problems in your spinal cord (which might make your legs go 'dead').

Treatment It's very unlikely that you'll have any of these problems. If you're concerned, see your GP.

Problems sleeping

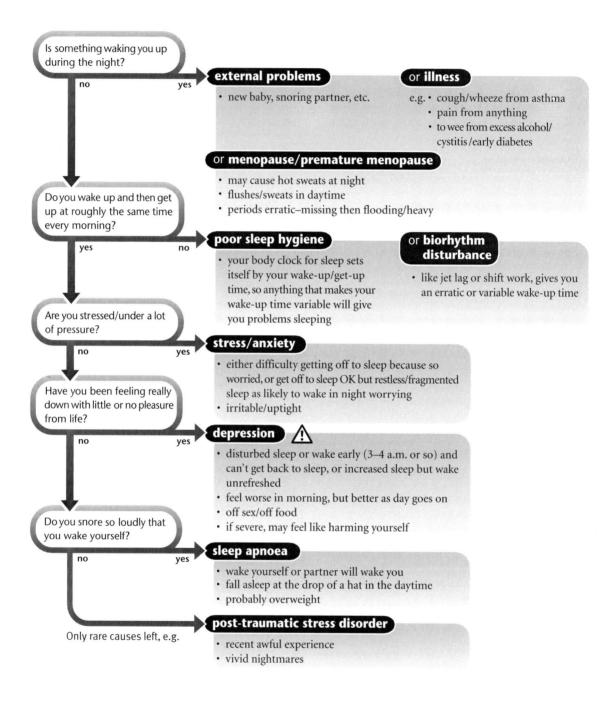

Is something waking you up during the night?
no / yes

external problems
- new baby, snoring partner, etc.

or illness
e.g. • cough/wheeze from asthma
- pain from anything
- to wee from excess alcohol/ cystitis/early diabetes

or menopause/premature menopause
- may cause hot sweats at night
- flushes/sweats in daytime
- periods erratic–missing then flooding/heavy

Do you wake up and then get up at roughly the same time every morning?
yes / no

poor sleep hygiene
- your body clock for sleep sets itself by your wake-up/get-up time, so anything that makes your wake-up time variable will give you problems sleeping

or biorhythm disturbance
- like jet lag or shift work, gives you an erratic or variable wake-up time

Are you stressed/under a lot of pressure?
no / yes

stress/anxiety
- either difficulty getting off to sleep because so worried, or get off to sleep OK but restless/fragmented sleep as likely to wake in night worrying
- irritable/uptight

Have you been feeling really down with little or no pleasure from life?
no / yes

depression ⚠
- disturbed sleep or wake early (3–4 a.m. or so) and can't get back to sleep, or increased sleep but wake unrefreshed
- feel worse in morning, but better as day goes on
- off sex/off food
- if severe, may feel like harming yourself

Do you snore so loudly that you wake yourself?
no / yes

sleep apnoea
- wake yourself or partner will wake you
- fall asleep at the drop of a hat in the daytime
- probably overweight

Only rare causes left, e.g.

post-traumatic stress disorder
- recent awful experience
- vivid nightmares

External problems Outside factors can stop you sleeping properly. These include being too cold or hot, the room not being dark enough, a snoring partner, or disturbances from your kids.

Treatment Getting your bedroom and bed as comfortable as possible will obviously help. Do this before you try to sleep rather than in the middle of the night. Wax ear plugs can help blot out the noise of a snoring partner. If your kids keep playing up at night, and so keeping you awake, check out one of the many books on taming your children, or discuss the problem with your health visitor (based at your GP's surgery).

Poor sleep hygiene Bad habits can mess up your sleep. These include too much caffeine (e.g. coffee, tea, and cola), regular alcohol, having an erratic routine, too much partying, illicit drugs, watching TV in bed, 'lying in' in the mornings, and taking naps during the day.

Treatment Sort out your lifestyle as best you can. A regular time for going to bed and waking, and avoiding dozing off during the day, are important. Exercising more will help. Don't try to zonk yourself out with booze, either – if used regularly, alcohol tends to disturb rather than help sleep. And in bed, don't toss and turn, watching the clock – if you really can't get to sleep, get up and do something for half an hour, then try again.

Stress and anxiety Feeling tense will make it hard for you to switch off, so you'll have trouble getting to sleep. You might also suffer from nightmares, which will aggravate the problem. The usual causes are worries about work, relationships, or money.

Treatment You'll find plenty of advice to help stress and anxiety in the 'Feeling tense' section (p.64) and the 'Anxiety' part of the 'Palpitations' section (p. 116). Increasing your exercise helps cut stress levels – sex, in particular is an excellent way of relaxing which will help you sleep properly. You might want to talk to your GP about the problem, but don't expect sleeping pills. These are rarely prescribed these days because they don't help that much and can be addictive if used for more than a few weeks. Sometimes they're useful just for a few days to break a cycle of bad sleep.

Depression Depression can disturb your sleep by making you wake earlier in the morning than you'd planned. For details, see the 'Feeling down' section (p.62).

Biorhythm disturbances Your body clock is usually set to follow the normal day/night pattern. It's not surprising, then, that messing it about – for example, through jet lag or shift work – will cause you problems sleeping.

Treatment If you're facing jet lag, make sure you don't drink too much booze on the plane, and sleep by your destination's time rather than by your body clock. Shift workers should set a regular sleep pattern, try to avoid being disturbed, and avoid the temptation to get up early to get things done during daylight hours. Sleeping tablets for a couple of days can occasionally be helpful in sorting out a biorhythm disturbance – discuss the situation with your GP.

Illness Various illnesses can disturb your sleep. These include any problem causing pain, asthma (if coughing or wheezing wake you), or waterworks problems.

Treatment The answer in this situation is to deal with the illness rather than the sleep problem – so speak to your GP.

Menopause/premature menopause The flushes and sweats which can occur during the menopause can be severe enough to disturb sleep. For more details, see the 'Flushing' section (p. 66).

Snoring/sleep apnoea Some people snore badly enough to disturb their own sleep, though this is more a problem in older age groups. A condition called 'sleep apnoea' causes earth-shattering snoring and can actually make you stop breathing for a short period in the night. You might regularly wake up coughing and spluttering and feel very dopey during the day. Your partner might tell you that your breathing seems to pack up in the night, or he might just leave you in disgust.

Treatment First, persuade your partner to try ear plugs. Next, slim down if you're overweight, and avoid alcohol late at night. If you're still in trouble, see your GP. There may be treatment to help, especially if you have sleep apnoea.

Post-traumatic stress disorder It's normal to have dreams or nightmares after an upsetting event. But if you've had some really awful experience, suffer vivid nightmares which disturb your sleep for more than a month and suffer other symptoms, you might have 'post-traumatic stress disorder' – a severe psychological reaction to an unpleasant event.

Treatment If the problem isn't getting better on its own, speak to your GP. She may treat you with antidepressants or refer you to a counsellor or psychiatrist.

Problems swallowing

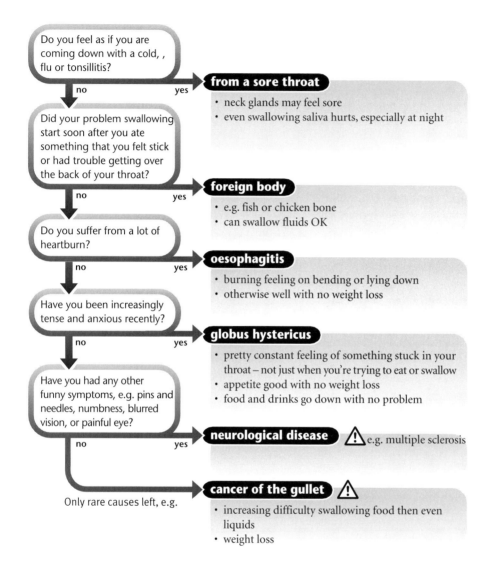

Do you feel as if you are coming down with a cold, , flu or tonsillitis?

no — yes →

from a sore throat
- neck glands may feel sore
- even swallowing saliva hurts, especially at night

Did your problem swallowing start soon after you ate something that you felt stick or had trouble getting over the back of your throat?

no — yes →

foreign body
- e.g. fish or chicken bone
- can swallow fluids OK

Do you suffer from a lot of heartburn?

no — yes →

oesophagitis
- burning feeling on bending or lying down
- otherwise well with no weight loss

Have you been increasingly tense and anxious recently?

no — yes →

globus hystericus
- pretty constant feeling of something stuck in your throat – not just when you're trying to eat or swallow
- appetite good with no weight loss
- food and drinks go down with no problem

Have you had any other funny symptoms, e.g. pins and needles, numbness, blurred vision, or painful eye?

no — yes →

neurological disease ⚠ e.g. multiple sclerosis

Only rare causes left, e.g.

cancer of the gullet ⚠
- increasing difficulty swallowing food then even liquids
- weight loss

Remember: ⚠ means see your GP sharpish; ⚠ means an urgent hospital job

Sore throat of any cause If your throat is sore, then obviously it's going to be painful to swallow. For full details of the possible causes and treatment, see the 'Sore throat' section (p. 136).

Foreign body A bone or jagged-edged food (such as a bolted-down bag of chips) can scratch the pharynx, causing pain on swallowing. More rarely, a piece of bone can get stuck in the throat or gullet, causing discomfort and difficulty swallowing.

Treatment A scratch will heal with no treatment in a few days. If you think a piece of bone has got stuck, try eating some bread and drinking plenty of water, which may succeed in shifting it. If it persists, your best bet is to go to casualty to get it sorted out.

Oesophagitis The stomach contains acid to help digest your food. A valve at the top of the stomach prevents this acid from rising up ('refluxing') into the gullet. Sometimes, this valve does not work properly, with the result that acid coats and inflames your gullet ('oesophagitis'). You may feel this as an unpleasant burning feeling in the centre of your chest, especially on bending over or lying down (this is known as heartburn). Sometimes you can even taste the acid in your mouth. The inflamed area of the gullet may swell, causing pain on swallowing and, sometimes, a feeling that food sticks for a few seconds before it passes into the stomach.

Treatment Quick and easy cures are available from the chemist. These include antacid tablets and liquids to coat the gullet and neutralize the acid, and more powerful acid suppressants. But it's worth looking at your lifestyle too, otherwise the problem will tend to come back again. Try cutting down on cigarettes, alcohol (especially binges), and spicy foods, and avoid acidic tablets like aspirin and ibuprofen. Shed some pounds if you're overweight, eat sensibly and regularly, and try to avoid having anything to eat or drink within a couple of hours of going to bed – this tends to open up the valve, letting acid reflux into your gullet while you sleep. If you do tend to wake at night with heartburn, you may be able to cure the problem simply by raising the head of your bed by a few inches (a couple of bricks under the legs of your bed at the head end will do the trick) so that you sleep on a slight slope with your head higher than your feet. Don't just prop yourself up with pillows – this can actually make it worse. If all else fails, see your GP who will be able to prescribe powerful acid suppressants.

Globus hystericus When you swallow, your food goes down a muscular funnel – the 'pharynx' – which channels it into the gullet. If you're feeling tense, the muscles of the pharynx can contract. This causes a sensation of something stuck in the throat ('globus hystericus') often described as feeling like an apple core. To get rid of this sensation, you'll tend to keep swallowing – unfortunately, this will make you focus on the symptom and may also make you worry that there is something seriously wrong. This, in turn, aggravates the tension and makes the symptom worse.

Treatment Half the battle is simply realizing that the symptom is caused by stress rather than anything sinister. This stops the vicious circle of tension causing the symptom causing more tension. Sorting out whatever in your life is getting you uptight is obviously important; making efforts to relax and taking some physical exercise will also help.

Neurological disease This means a disease of the nervous system (which controls and coordinates the body's sensation and movements). Diseases of this sort can affect the body in many ways, including how the muscles of the gullet coordinate and whether or not the valve at the entrance to the stomach opens properly. There are many different types and, fortunately, they're all very rare.

Treatment If your GP shares your concern, she'll refer you for tests.

Cancer Gullet cancer is very rare in the under 50s. Cancers of the lymph glands, which can cause trouble swallowing by pressing on the gullet, are more common, but highly unlikely to reveal themselves just with this particular symptom.

Treatment Discuss your symptoms with your GP, who will arrange any necessary tests or specialist appointments.

Problems with sexual intercourse

NB If your problem is that you have gone off sex, see the specific 'Loss of sex drive' section (p. 90).

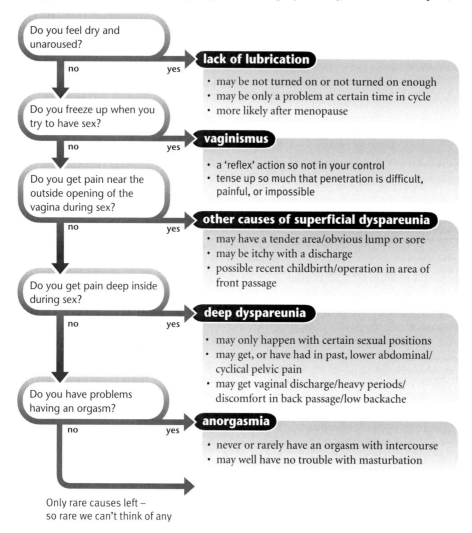

Do you feel dry and unaroused?
no / yes

lack of lubrication
- may be not turned on or not turned on enough
- may be only a problem at certain time in cycle
- more likely after menopause

Do you freeze up when you try to have sex?
no / yes

vaginismus
- a 'reflex' action so not in your control
- tense up so much that penetration is difficult, painful, or impossible

Do you get pain near the outside opening of the vagina during sex?
no / yes

other causes of superficial dyspareunia
- may have a tender area/obvious lump or sore
- may be itchy with a discharge
- possible recent childbirth/operation in area of front passage

Do you get pain deep inside during sex?
no / yes

deep dyspareunia
- may only happen with certain sexual positions
- may get, or have had in past, lower abdominal/cyclical pelvic pain
- may get vaginal discharge/heavy periods/discomfort in back passage/low backache

Do you have problems having an orgasm?
no / yes

anorgasmia
- never or rarely have an orgasm with intercourse
- may well have no trouble with masturbation

Only rare causes left –
so rare we can't think of any

Lack of lubrication During sexual excitement, glands around the front passage (the vagina) produce a natural lubricant. The amount of fluid, and the ease with which it appears, varies from woman to woman. If there's not much lubricant produced – for example, if you're not sufficiently aroused – then penetration can be difficult and uncomfortable.

Treatment If the problem lies in inadequate stimulation, then you really need to discuss the situation with your partner. Maybe he needs to concentrate more on foreplay. Or maybe he's simply not pressing the right buttons to turn you on. There are plenty of books and videos on the subject to help him. Another cause is anxiety – if you're uptight then you're unlikely to relax enough to become 'turned on' and this will prevent natural lubrication. In this situation, the answer lies in sorting out whatever is worrying you. Alternatively, it may be that you simply produce little of your own natural lubricant. This can easily be sorted out using KY jelly during sex or by suggesting imaginative use of a natural lubricant – his saliva.

Vaginismus This is a spasm of the muscles around the entrance to the vagina which occurs during attempted sex. The cause is thought to be a 'fear' of penetration, which makes you feel as though your vagina is too small to cope with the insertion of a penis. A vicious circle develops: attempted penetration is difficult and painful so that, next time, you'll be anxious, so there is little natural lubrication and lots of muscle spasm, which aggravates the problem.

Treatment It's worth working on relaxation exercises so that you learn how to stop your muscles tensing up. A little alcohol can be an effective relaxant, although it's sensible not to rely on this long term. Also, it's important to get any fears or hang-ups about sex out in the open with your partner. But there are also some self-help steps which can improve the situation. The first stage involves learning how to examine yourself. When lying in the bath, feeling relaxed, try gently putting one of your fingers into your vagina just a short way. Next bath time, try inserting it a little further. If you manage to avoid tensing up, you'll be surprised how roomy your vagina feels. Gradually build up your confidence, until you can put two fingers inside. The next step is to encourage your partner to insert his fingers in the same way, while you concentrate on staying relaxed. You'll soon realize that you could easily accommodate his penis. It's then a natural progression to full intercourse. If you get nowhere with this technique your GP may be able to help further, or she may refer you both to a psychosexual counsellor (a 'sexpert' skilled at dealing with this type of problem).

Other causes of superficial dyspareunia Superficial dyspareunia is the medical term for painful sex caused by something on or near the outside of the opening of your vagina (the 'vulva'). Two common causes – inadequate lubrication and vaginismus – are described above. There are a number of other possible causes, including infections such as thrush, scars (from tears or episiotomies during childbirth), and atrophic vaginitis, which is the thinning of the vaginal skin occurring after the menopause.

Treatment Thrush and other infections are dealt with in the 'Vaginal discharge' (p. 148) and 'Vulval irritation and/or sores' (p. 158) sections; the latter section also discusses atrophic vaginitis. If the problem is caused by a scar and is showing no signs of improving with time, then you should discuss the situation with your GP.

Anorgasmia This means inability to have an orgasm. It may be that you've never had an orgasm, or that you have problems achieving a climax during sex with your partner while you manage fine when you mastubate. There are usually a number of factors involved – not least the impression given through the media that sex is only satisfactory if it always ends with a monumental orgasm. If it is a real problem then it will probably involve, on the woman's side, a failure to relax and 'let go', and on the man's side, poor sexual knowledge or technique. Repeated 'failure' leads to frustration and dejection on both sides, which makes the problem worse. Of course, it could simply be that you're not attracted to your partner – or to men in general!

Treatment The media pressure to have perfect sex is unrealistic. If you're both happy with your sex life, even if you don't climax often, then you needn't worry. On the other hand, if you're dissatisfied with your ability to reach orgasm, there is plenty that can be achieved. It's important to learn to relax so that you can 'let go' during sex, and any sexual hang-ups or relationship problems should be brought out into the open. You might let him know how you turn yourself on when you masturbate so that he can try these 'tricks' himself. 'Learning' how to masturbate may prove very helpful if you've never been able to reach orgasm. Other practical tips include getting your partner to bring you very close to orgasm before he penetrates you with his penis. If all else fails, discuss the situation with your GP, who may refer you both to a psychosexual counsellor.

Deep dyspareunia This means pain deep inside during sex. There are a number of causes, including 'collision dyspareunia' (which means simply that the natural arrangement of your womb and ovaries in your pelvis results in them being 'bashed' by your partner's penis during sex – and so only occurs in certain positions), chronic pelvic inflammatory disease, and endometriosis.

Treatment Collision dyspareunia can usually be solved by experimenting with different positions for sex; chronic pelvic inflammatory disease and endometriosis are discussed in the 'Abdominal pain – recurrent' section (p. 10). Unless it's clear that your problem is due to collision dyspareunia, a trip to your GP is advisable so that she can check you out for possible serious rarities like an ovarian cyst.

Is your rash mainly on your face, very itchy, or made up of blisters?

no — yes ►

turn to
- 'Rash on the face' p.128
- 'Itchy skin'   p.84
- 'Blisters'   p.30

Have you been unwell with a sore throat, temperature, aches or have you been in contact with someone with a rash?

no — yes ►

virus
- in most cases rash will be flat red spots or spots that are slightly raised
- rash may be first or only sign of a virus infection

Is your rash in obvious patches, i.e. well marked out from rest of skin?

no — yes ►

eczema
- skin dry/red, sometimes with itchy small blisters
- if gets weepy, may be a sign that it's infected
- may be an allergy, e.g. to metal or cosmetics
- may get repeated attacks

or pregnancy
- may cause purplish stretch marks on tummy
- may cause dark brown marks round nipple/belly button

or psoriasis
- thick, red, scaly plaques of skin, especially on elbows/knees/scalp
- may be a long-term problem

or fungal infections
- may be under armpit; on body (ringworm); in groin; or on feet (athlete's foot)
- skin dry and red with redness most obvious at edge of infected area, though in groin or toes may be moist with skin cracked

Is the rash over most of your body?

no — yes ►

allergy to medication
- especially antibiotics like penicillin
- dramatic onset of rash/may feel ill, have a temperature
- if like nettle rash, most often from antibiotics
- if like measles (widespread red, slightly raised spots), most often from amoxycillin, anti-rheumatic drugs
- most serious kind will blister and erode the skin ⚠

or pregnancy
- may cause rashes, especially later on in pregnancy – likely to be itchy

or pityriasis rosea
- one patch appears on body before rest
- oval, scaly, pink patches, each 2 cm or so in diameter
- tend to be arranged around the trunk in the lines of the ribs

or eczema ⚠
- which may suddenly become widespread

or psoriasis ⚠
- small, scaly spots over body after sore throat
- may suddenly worsen with redness/scaling spreading over body – may make you very ill

Only rare skin problems or unusual forms of common problems left

 Very rarely, a rash may be caused by meningitis. The small red spots do not blanch (go white) under pressure and spread rapidly. By the time the spots appear, you are likely to be seriously ill.

Virus A rash is just one of the many symptoms (like fever and sore throat) that a virus produces as it works its way through your system.

Treatment There's no magic cure for a virus. Try paracetamol if you feel hot and achy, and calamine lotion if the rash is itchy. It usually disappears after a few days. It's worth seeking the advice of your GP if you're pregnant – although most viruses cause the baby no problem, especially once you're past the early stages of pregnancy, a few can cause trouble. For this reason, it's also a good idea to steer clear of women who are (or might be) pregnant until you're better. For more information about chickenpox and shingles – caused by one particular type of virus – see the 'Blisters' section (p. 30).

Eczema/dermatitis This is explained, and the treatment outlined, in the 'Itchy skin' section (p. 84).

Psoriasis The layers of your skin usually replace themselves every month. If you have psoriasis, your skin for some reason goes into overdrive, causing patches of thickening and scaling. It sometimes runs in families.

Treatment Like eczema, patches may come and go or it may affect your skin constantly. Moisturizers and creams or lotions containing coal tar can help (available from the chemist). See your GP if you're getting nowhere as there are lots of other effective treatments – and if necessary, she can refer you to a dermatologist (skin specialist).

Fungal infections Athlete's foot is an infection caused by a fungus. Similar infections can occur on other areas of the skin, especially where it's moist, such as the armpit or groin.

Treatment Keep the areas clean and dry and get an antifungal cream from the chemist. If this doesn't work, see your GP.

Pityriasis rosea This is quite common, especially in adolescents and young adults in autumn and winter. It is possibly due to a virus, although it's not infectious.

Treatment No treatment is needed – it goes away on its own, though it may take a few weeks. If it's a bit irritating, try a moisturizer from the chemist.

Allergy to medication Any medication – prescribed or over the counter – can cause an allergic rash, but the most likely culprits are antibiotics, aspirin, or anti-inflammatory drugs like ibuprofen. The type of rash varies, but it can be 'urticaria' (see the 'Itchy skin' section, p. 00). You might not make the connection between the rash and the medication – you may have taken the treatment before without any problem, or the rash may take three weeks from the first dose to appear.

Treatment Stop the treatment which has caused the rash and don't take it again. Also, let your doctor know what has happened (just leave her a message) so the allergy goes on your medical records. The rash usually goes within a few days. If you have urticaria, take the advice given in the 'Urticaria' part of the 'Itchy skin' section (p. 84).

Rashes caused by pregnancy Pregnancy commonly results in stretch marks and a darkening of some pigmented skin areas (such as around the nipples). But some other unusual and very itchy skin problems can be caused by the hormone changes that occur in pregnancy.

Treatment You'll need to see your GP to confirm the cause of the rash. Then it's usually just a case of using moisturizers or calamine lotion to ease the problem, which will go once you've had the baby. Very occasionally, if the rash is very itchy, you might need blood tests or even treatment by a dermatologist. Some of these problems come back in future pregnancies and some don't – your doctor should be able to advise you.

Unusual skin problems There are a number of rare skin problems. Also, the rashes of even the more common skin diseases are sometimes not typical. An odd, reddish rash which doesn't blanch (in other words, fade when pressed with a glass), especially if you feel unwell at the same time (with, for example, a headache, fever, or vomiting), just might be the very rare 'meningitis rash'.

Treatment If you really think there is a chance you might have the meningitis rash, you're probably wrong, but seek medical advice immediately to be sure. Otherwise, book an appointment to check out your rash with your GP. If she's stuck for an answer and it's a nuisance to you, she'll probably refer you to a dermatologist.

Rash on the face

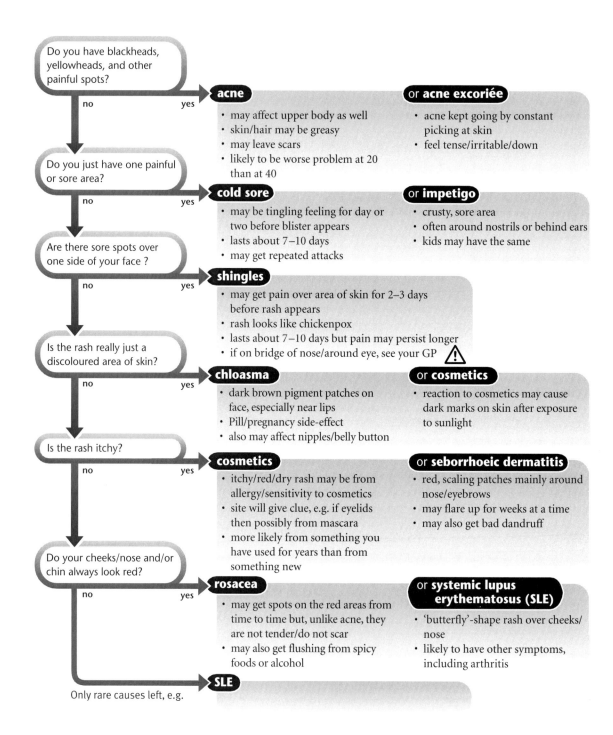

Do you have blackheads, yellowheads, and other painful spots?

no / yes

acne
- may affect upper body as well
- skin/hair may be greasy
- may leave scars
- likely to be worse problem at 20 than at 40

or acne excoriée
- acne kept going by constant picking at skin
- feel tense/irritable/down

Do you just have one painful or sore area?

no / yes

cold sore
- may be tingling feeling for day or two before blister appears
- lasts about 7–10 days
- may get repeated attacks

or impetigo
- crusty, sore area
- often around nostrils or behind ears
- kids may have the same

Are there sore spots over one side of your face ?

no / yes

shingles
- may get pain over area of skin for 2–3 days before rash appears
- rash looks like chickenpox
- lasts about 7–10 days but pain may persist longer
- if on bridge of nose/around eye, see your GP ⚠

Is the rash really just a discoloured area of skin?

no / yes

chloasma
- dark brown pigment patches on face, especially near lips
- Pill/pregnancy side-effect
- also may affect nipples/belly button

or cosmetics
- reaction to cosmetics may cause dark marks on skin after exposure to sunlight

Is the rash itchy?

no / yes

cosmetics
- itchy/red/dry rash may be from allergy/sensitivity to cosmetics
- site will give clue, e.g. if eyelids then possibly from mascara
- more likely from something you have used for years than from something new

or seborrhoeic dermatitis
- red, scaling patches mainly around nose/eyebrows
- may flare up for weeks at a time
- may also get bad dandruff

Do your cheeks/nose and/or chin always look red?

no / yes

rosacea
- may get spots on the red areas from time to time but, unlike acne, they are not tender/do not scar
- may also get flushing from spicy foods or alcohol

or systemic lupus erythematosus (SLE)
- 'butterfly'-shape rash over cheeks/nose
- likely to have other symptoms, including arthritis

SLE

Only rare causes left, e.g.

Rash on the face

Acne This is very common and is, to some extent, a normal part of adolescence. It may not disappear until your mid 20s and sometimes develops in older age groups. It's caused by the glands which produce the normal grease on your skin getting blocked. This results in 'blackheads', and infection of the stagnant grease leads to the inflamed pus spots characteristic of acne. When very severe, it can cause large cysts and scarring.

Treatment Mild acne needs no treatment at all if it doesn't bother you. Getting out in the sunshine helps, but altering your diet won't make any difference. It's important to keep your skin clean to remove excess grease and reduce the germs which aggravate the problem. You'll find some effective treatments available over the counter: for example, benzoyl peroxide (cream, gel, or lotion). If this doesn't work, or your acne is severe – especially if you're getting cysts or scarring – see your GP. She can prescribe a number of effective treatments (such as antibiotics) and, if they don't work, or your acne is really bad, she may refer you to a dermatologist (skin specialist) for more powerful treatment.

Seborrhoeic dermatitis The cause is thought to be an infection with a fungus. The rash can affect other areas, such as your scalp, chest, groin, and armpits.

Treatment You should be able to sort this out using an anti-fungal cream (such as clotrimazole, available from the chemist), which is perfectly safe to use on the face. The rash can come back – just use the cream when you need to. If the scalp is affected, it's important to clear that up too by using an anti-fungal shampoo regularly (see the 'Itchy scalp' section, p. 82).

Cold sore This is caused by a virus (the herpes simplex virus). Once you've had an attack, the virus lies dormant in a nerve and can reactivate at certain times, resulting in repeated attacks, nearly always in the same area (usually the lip). There may be no particular trigger for attacks but stress, periods, being run down, and sunlight may bring them on.

Treatment There is no 'cure' to get rid of the virus once and for all. Some people find that using a cream from the chemist – aciclovir – at the first sign of an attack can help a little.

Cosmetics Cosmetics can cause problems in two different ways. First, they can cause an allergic reaction – often, the allergy is linked to something you've been using a long time rather than something new. Second, they can increase the pigment in your skin, causing dark marks, especially after exposure to sunlight.

Treatment Obviously, it's important to stop using the cosmetic which is causing the problem – this is often a case of trial and error. If the rash it has caused is very itchy, you can settle it down with hydrocortisone 1% cream (available from the chemist). Any excess pigmentation the cosmetic

has caused should fade, though this may take months.

Chloasma This is linked with hormones – pregnancy or the Pill can occasionally increase the amount of pigment, in patches, on your face.

Treatment The problem often goes when you've had your baby or stopped the Pill. Use a sunscreen on your face when exposed to sunlight, otherwise the pigment will darken. There is no really effective treatment for this condition.

Acne excoriée Whatever starts this problem in the first place – and it's often just a simple attack of mild acne – it's kept going by constant picking of the skin. It's usually linked with tension or depression, and a vicious cycle develops: if you're tense or down, you may become preoccupied with your appearance so you tend to pick your spots more, which makes it worse, causing further emotional upset.

Treatment The key point is to leave your face alone, which may not be easy as you're likely to be quite obsessed with the problem. No amount of cream or lotions will help and may actually make matters worse. If you do feel very stressed or depressed then it's probably more constructive to focus on this than your skin – see the 'Feeling down' (p. 62) or 'Feeling tense' (p. 64) sections.

Rosacea The cause for this combination of pus spots, redness, and flushing is unknown. It usually starts in your 40s.

Treatment Alcohol, hot drinks, and spicy foods can aggravate the flushing, so you may want to avoid, or cut down, these. Otherwise, there's not much you can do in the way of self-treatment. If the problem is a real nuisance, see your GP, as she can prescribe effective treatment such as antibiotic creams or tablets.

Shingles This is explained, and the treatment discussed, in the 'Blisters' section (p. 30). If you think you're developing shingles on the face, especially if it's near the eye, you need to see your GP within a day or two – and urgently if the eyeball itself is red or sore.

(**Impetigo**) This is an infection of the skin by a germ. It may get into the skin through a cut or graze, or it may infect eczema or a cold sore.

Treatment A mild attack may be sorted out with an antiseptic cream. Otherwise, you'll need to see your GP for antibiotics.

(**Rare skin problems**) Occasionally, rashes on the face can be linked with some other problem, such as certain types of arthritis (one example being systemic lupus erythematosus, or 'SLE').

Treatment It's unlikely that you have one of these unusual conditions. If you're concerned, and especially if you have joint pain and swellings too, see your GP. If she thinks it necessary, she'll refer you to a skin or joint specialist.

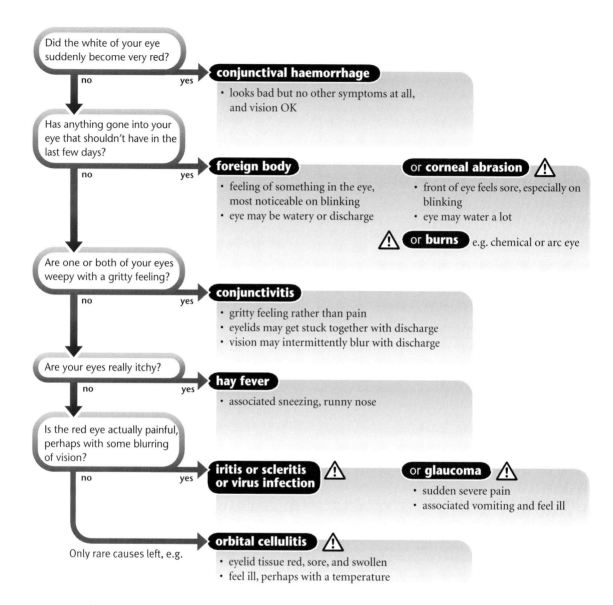

Did the white of your eye suddenly become very red?
— no / yes →

conjunctival haemorrhage
- looks bad but no other symptoms at all, and vision OK

Has anything gone into your eye that shouldn't have in the last few days?
— no / yes →

foreign body
- feeling of something in the eye, most noticeable on blinking
- eye may be watery or discharge

or corneal abrasion ⚠
- front of eye feels sore, especially on blinking
- eye may water a lot

⚠ **or burns** e.g. chemical or arc eye

Are one or both of your eyes weepy with a gritty feeling?
— no / yes →

conjunctivitis
- gritty feeling rather than pain
- eyelids may get stuck together with discharge
- vision may intermittently blur with discharge

Are your eyes really itchy?
— no / yes →

hay fever
- associated sneezing, runny nose

Is the red eye actually painful, perhaps with some blurring of vision?
— no / yes →

iritis or scleritis or virus infection ⚠

or glaucoma ⚠
- sudden severe pain
- associated vomiting and feel ill

Only rare causes left, e.g.

orbital cellulitis ⚠
- eyelid tissue red, sore, and swollen
- feel ill, perhaps with a temperature

Remember: ⚠ means see your GP sharpish; ⚠ means an urgent hospital job

Conjunctivitis The eye has a delicate cling-film wrapper type covering: the conjunctiva. When this gets infected, usually from a cold, it becomes reddened and discharges mucky pus – this is conjunctivitis.

Treatment A mild, early case can be cured with gentle, regular bathing of the eye using cotton wool soaked in warm water. If it's not getting any better, or the eyes are really sticky and sore, see your GP for some antibiotic eye ointment.

Hay fever Allergy to pollen causes hay fever. The eyes alone may be affected, or they may just be part of the overall runny nosed, sneezing misery.

Treatment Simple measures include avoiding long walks when the pollen count is high (usually early morning and evening), wearing sunglasses to reduce glare, and keeping the car windows wound up (otherwise the car acts as a pollen trap). It's worth a trip to the chemist: various eye-drops, or antihistamine tablets, can help a lot.

Foreign body A bit of dirt or debris on the eye or under the lids will cause irritation.

Treatment If something has simply blown into the eye, get someone to gently remove it with the corner of a hanky. There are a couple of tricks you can use to sort out something caught under the upper lid. Try turning the lid inside out – you can do this by grasping the eyelashes in one hand, and using a cotton bud in the other to gently push on the upper surface of the lid, rolling the lid around the bud. Your accomplice should now be able to fish out the offending piece of dirt. If you're on your own, try pulling the upper lid down, by the lashes, over the lower lid, then releasing. As the upper lid returns to its normal position, the lower lid lashes may sift out the foreign body. Tiny pieces of metal from grinding can stick on the front of the eye or even enter the eye itself. Get it checked at casualty.

Corneal abrasion A scratch on the front of the eye. This is usually caused by a minor injury – like from a twig or a baby's fingernail – or a foreign body (see above).

Treatment See your GP. She will assess the damage and probably treat you with antibiotic ointment. If it doesn't heal quickly – usually within a day or two – you may need to see an eye specialist.

Conjunctival haemorrhage A leak of blood in the conjunctiva. It usually appears for no obvious reason, but may be caused by violent coughing or retching.

Treatment Despite its dramatic appearance, it needs no treatment at all – it's perfectly harmless and disappears within a few days.

Iritis Inflammation of the coloured part of the eye (the iris). It is sometimes connected to rare types of arthritis.

Treatment See your GP – she'll probably send you to an eye specialist urgently to get it checked out and for treatment with eye drops. The problem can recur: your specialist is likely to tell you what action to take should you get further problems.

Burns Chemicals splashed into the eye can result in burns. So too can very bright light, such as the 'dazzle' from arc welding – if you go in for that sort of thing and you don't wear goggles, it can cause a flash burn.

Treatment If a chemical has splashed into your eye, wash it out with lots of water, then go to casualty for further treatment (try to take the name of the chemical with you). For arc eye, see your GP for treatment with drops – and wear goggles in future.

Virus infection Herpes simplex is the virus which causes cold sores. Rarely, it can infect the eye, causing ulcers and inflammation. Shingles is caused by a similar virus and can also affect the eye (see the 'Blisters' section, p. 30, for more details).

Treatment Another GP job and likely to need urgent specialist treatment if confirmed.

Scleritis Inflammation of the white of the eye. Like iritis, it can be linked to joint problems (such as rheumatoid arthritis).

Treatment Check with your GP – you're likely to need to see an eye specialist.

Orbital cellulitis An infection of the hole – the orbit – in which the eye sits, which usually then spreads to the eye itself.

Treatment Can get very nasty if not treated quickly with antibiotics. See your GP, who may send you to hospital.

Acute glaucoma A sudden increase in the pressure of the fluid in the eye. Very rare in the under 50s.

Treatment If your GP thinks you have got acute glaucoma, which is pretty unlikely, she'll send you straight to the eye specialist.

Shortness of breath

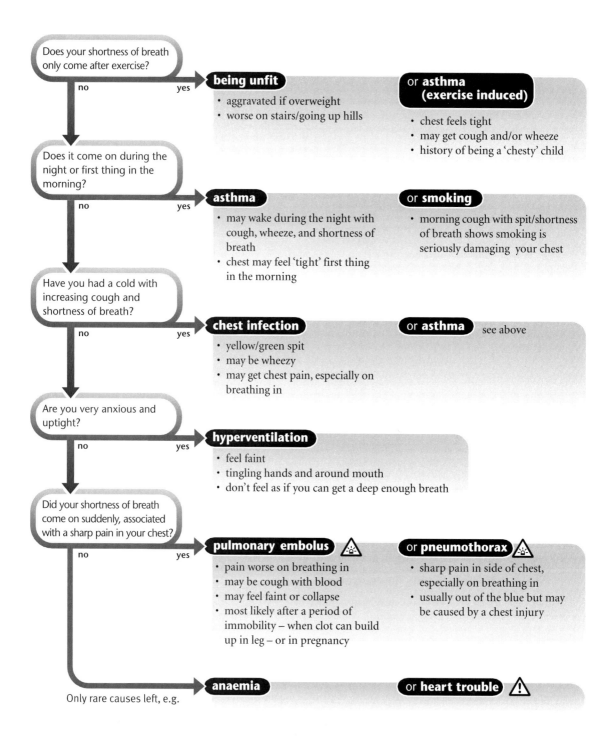

Does your shortness of breath only come after exercise?

no → yes →

being unfit
- aggravated if overweight
- worse on stairs/going up hills

or **asthma (exercise induced)**
- chest feels tight
- may get cough and/or wheeze
- history of being a 'chesty' child

Does it come on during the night or first thing in the morning?

no → yes →

asthma
- may wake during the night with cough, wheeze, and shortness of breath
- chest may feel 'tight' first thing in the morning

or **smoking**
- morning cough with spit/shortness of breath shows smoking is seriously damaging your chest

Have you had a cold with increasing cough and shortness of breath?

no → yes →

chest infection
- yellow/green spit
- may be wheezy
- may get chest pain, especially on breathing in

or **asthma** see above

Are you very anxious and uptight?

no → yes →

hyperventilation
- feel faint
- tingling hands and around mouth
- don't feel as if you can get a deep enough breath

Did your shortness of breath come on suddenly, associated with a sharp pain in your chest?

no → yes →

pulmonary embolus
- pain worse on breathing in
- may be cough with blood
- may feel faint or collapse
- most likely after a period of immobility – when clot can build up in leg – or in pregnancy

or **pneumothorax**
- sharp pain in side of chest, especially on breathing in
- usually out of the blue but may be caused by a chest injury

anaemia

or **heart trouble**

Only rare causes left, e.g.

Shortness of breath

Being unfit and/or overweight If you've let yourself get out of shape, you're bound to feel more short of breath than usual after you've run up a few flights of stairs. You'll notice it even more if you're overweight, simply because you're effectively carrying excess baggage around all the time.

Treatment Get fit. Break yourself back in gently, though – if you launch into frenzied aerobics from the start you risk injuring yourself or making yourself ill. Gradually improve your level of fitness and aim for about three sessions of exercise of around half an hour each week (enough to make you sweat). This will help you shed excess pounds too, as will a revamp of your diet.

Smoking Everyone knows that cigarette smoke can permanently damage the lungs and aggravate other lung conditions (such as asthma – see below). It also lowers the levels of oxygen in the blood, narrows the airways, and reduces the volume of your lungs.

Treatment Cut down, and preferably give up, the ciggies. Only do this when you feel really motivated because otherwise you'll fail which may make you believe you can never succeed. Get as much help as you can – read a leaflet or book on how to give up, persuade your partner to stop too, and get all cigarettes and ashtrays out of the house. Make sure the Big Day is during a phase when you're not too stressed, and then just stop – don't mess around trying to wean yourself off them. Staying stopped is the really tricky bit. Avoid situations which prompt you to have a fag, and consider using nicotine replacement (available from the chemist as a gum, patch, or nose spray) or tablets like Zyban (from your GP) if you get really bad cravings. You're very likely to need nicotine treatment or tablets if you light up first thing in the morning or smoke more than 20 a day. And don't worry if you put on weight – you can sort that out once you're over the ciggies. Most people who manage to give up do so with simple advice and maybe nicotine replacement treatment. A few use other measures such as hypnotherapy, but you may be better off taking a long hard look at why you've failed to give up, and trying to put it right, than spending money on a miracle cure. If you don't *really* want to stop, then no treatment on earth is going to help you kick the habit.

Asthma This is explained, and the treatment discussed, in the 'Cough' section (p. 46).

Chest infection See the 'Cough' section (p. 46).

Hyperventilation If you don't think you're getting enough air into your lungs, you'll tend to breathe deeper or faster – this is hyperventilation. It is usually caused by anxiety because tension tends to tighten up the muscles of the rib cage so that you feel your chest isn't expanding enough. A vicious cycle builds up because the feeling of breathlessness increases the anxiety, tensing up the muscles even more. A sudden, severe attack is known as a 'panic attack'.

Treatment Try to get to the root of the problem by sorting out the main stresses in your life. Relaxation therapy can help (whatever switches you off) and physical exercise will also burn off nervous energy. A panic attack can be helped by making sure that those around you know what's going on (otherwise they'll panic too, making you worse), trying to stay calm, and breathing in and out of a paper bag. If you seem to be getting nowhere, see your GP – she may be able to sort out anxiety management sessions for you. Very occasionally, you might need medication, especially if your hyperventilation is a part of depression (see the 'Feeling down' section, p 62).

Pulmonary embolus This is a blood clot on the lung. It usually starts in the legs (a 'deep vein thrombosis') and can make the calf swollen and painful – see the 'Calf pain' section (p. 42). This clot can then travel up to the lung. It's usually linked to being immobile – for example, being in a plaster because of a broken leg – and is a bit more common in pregnant women and in women who use the Pill, especially if they smoke.

Treatment A clot on the lung requires urgent hospital attention. You'll need to avoid the Pill in the future as this increases the risk of another one.

Pneumothorax This is a collapsed lung. Air suddenly escapes into the gap between the lung and the ribs, squashing the lung. It usually happens for no particular reason, though it can be caused by an injury such as a broken rib or a stab wound.

Treatment If you think you might have a pneumothorax, your best bet is to go straight to casualty.

Other medical conditions A whole heap of other problems can cause breathlessness. These include anaemia, heart valve problems, chronic bronchitis, and angina. Fortunately, none are likely to apply to you.

Treatment In less 'urgent' situations, make an appointment with your GP. However, if the shortness of breath is sudden and severe, go straight to hospital.

Skin marks and lumps

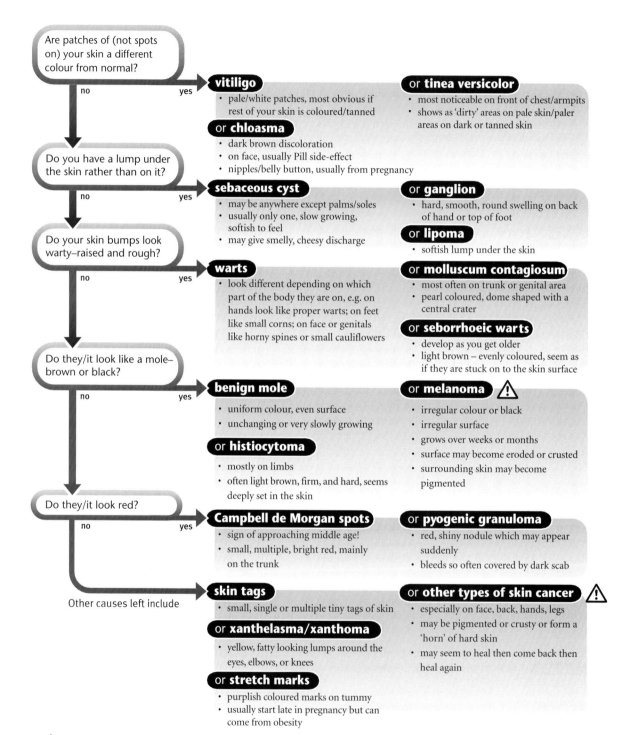

Are patches of (not spots on) your skin a different colour from normal?

no / yes

vitiligo
- pale/white patches, most obvious if rest of your skin is coloured/tanned

or chloasma
- dark brown discoloration
- on face, usually Pill side-effect
- nipples/belly button, usually from pregnancy

or tinea versicolor
- most noticeable on front of chest/armpits
- shows as 'dirty' areas on pale skin/paler areas on dark or tanned skin

Do you have a lump under the skin rather than on it?

no / yes

sebaceous cyst
- may be anywhere except palms/soles
- usually only one, slow growing, softish to feel
- may give smelly, cheesy discharge

or ganglion
- hard, smooth, round swelling on back of hand or top of foot

or lipoma
- softish lump under the skin

Do your skin bumps look warty–raised and rough?

no / yes

warts
- look different depending on which part of the body they are on, e.g. on hands look like proper warts; on feet like small corns; on face or genitals like horny spines or small cauliflowers

or molluscum contagiosum
- most often on trunk or genital area
- pearl coloured, dome shaped with a central crater

or seborrhoeic warts
- develop as you get older
- light brown – evenly coloured, seem as if they are stuck on to the skin surface

Do they/it look like a mole–brown or black?

no / yes

benign mole
- uniform colour, even surface
- unchanging or very slowly growing

or histiocytoma
- mostly on limbs
- often light brown, firm, and hard, seems deeply set in the skin

or melanoma ⚠
- irregular colour or black
- irregular surface
- grows over weeks or months
- surface may become eroded or crusted
- surrounding skin may become pigmented

Do they/it look red?

no / yes

Campbell de Morgan spots
- sign of approaching middle age!
- small, multiple, bright red, mainly on the trunk

or pyogenic granuloma
- red, shiny nodule which may appear suddenly
- bleeds so often covered by dark scab

Other causes left include

skin tags
- small, single or multiple tiny tags of skin

or xanthelasma/xanthoma
- yellow, fatty looking lumps around the eyes, elbows, or knees

or stretch marks
- purplish coloured marks on tummy
- usually start late in pregnancy but can come from obesity

or other types of skin cancer ⚠
- especially on face, back, hands, legs
- may be pigmented or crusty or form a 'horn' of hard skin
- may seem to heal then come back then heal again

⚠ Any coloured skin mark which is changing colour or size, or which bleeds easily, should be checked by a doctor.

Skin marks and lumps

Benign moles Little clusters of the cells in the skin which produce pigment.

Treatment They can be left alone but need to be distinguished from 'melanoma' (see the flow chart).

Warts/molluscum contagiosum (NB *For information about warts on the genitals, see the 'Vulval irritation and/or sores' section*) Warts are caused by a virus and can occur anywhere, especially on the hands and feet (where they're known as verrucas). Molluscum contagiosum are similar, and are also caused by a virus. If they appear on your genitals or lower abdomen, they may have been passed on sexually.

Treatment Warts eventually go on their own, although they can take years. If you want to get rid of them, use a lotion from the chemist to soften the skin, then rub with a pumice stone – but this may take weeks to work. If you're really desperate, see your GP, who might arrange to have them frozen off. Genital warts need special assessment and treatment (see the 'Vulval irritation and/or sores' section). Molluscum contagiosum go on their own eventually. You can speed things up by pricking them with a sterile needle – or you can see your GP, who might freeze them off.

Skin tags Tiny extra flaps of skin. What causes them is unknown.

Treatment These can be left alone. If you want to get rid of them, see your GP.

Sebaceous cyst If one of the glands which produces the grease on your skin gets blocked, the grease can't escape and so forms a lump – a sebaceous cyst.

Treatment These are harmless and so don't need any treatment. A cyst can be removed if it's a nuisance – see your GP, who will sort it out (a very simple minor operation).

Campbell de Morgan spots Numerous small red spots which develop in your late 30s or early 40s.

Treatment None required as they're completely normal.

Chloasma This is explained in the 'Rash on the face' section (p. 128).

Vitiligo This makes the pigment-producing cells of your skin pack up. The cause is unknown, and it sometimes runs in families.

Treatment Unfortunately, most people with vitiligo are stuck with it. Many of the treatments tried don't achieve much, though you may want to discuss this with your GP. It's important to use sunblocks in the summer – the problem will look much worse if your 'normal' skin tans. Camouflage cosmetics can help a lot if you're desperate.

Ganglion A hard, fluid-filled lump which develops over a joint. The cause is unknown.

Treatment They're safe to leave alone. They can be cut out, but it's not a small operation and it might come back.

Lipoma A fatty lump under the skin, cause unknown.

Treatment It's safe to leave well alone.

Seborrhoeic warts A warty overgrowth of skin. They're much commoner in the elderly, but they can occur in younger age groups.

Treatment Totally harmless; they can be frozen off if they're a nuisance.

Stretch marks Lines of stretched skin, usually on the lower part of your abdomen. They're caused mainly by pregnancy or being overweight.

Treatment These are permanent – there's no effective treatment for them.

Xanthelasma/xanthoma Collections of fat (xanthelasma occurs around the eyes and xanthoma on the elbows or knees). They are sometimes caused by a high cholesterol level in your blood.

Treatment None is needed, but it's worth getting your cholesterol level checked.

Pyogenic granuloma A small skin lump, probably caused by a very minor injury.

Treatment See your GP to get it checked and, if necessary, removed.

Tinea versicolor An infection with a type of fungus.

Treatment Anti-fungal creams from the chemist will usually cure the problem, but you may need to use them for a few weeks. Selenium sulphide shampoo (available over the counter) can also help. Apply once a week for eight weeks, then wash it off after a few hours. Use it on your scalp too, as the fungus may live in your hair and then reinfect your skin. This rash can cause patches of your skin to lighten – this can take months to improve, even after treatment.

Melanoma This is a skin cancer developing from the cells which produce pigment – it can sometimes start in a mole. The cause is thought to be exposure to sunlight (especially severe episodes of sunburn in childhood) and, in women, it's commonest on the legs.

Treatment See your GP asap. If she thinks you might have a melanoma, she'll refer you to a dermatologist (skin specialist).

Other skin cancers These are unusual in the under 45s and, again, are probably linked to sun exposure.

Treatment See your GP, who will refer you to a dermatologist.

Sore throat

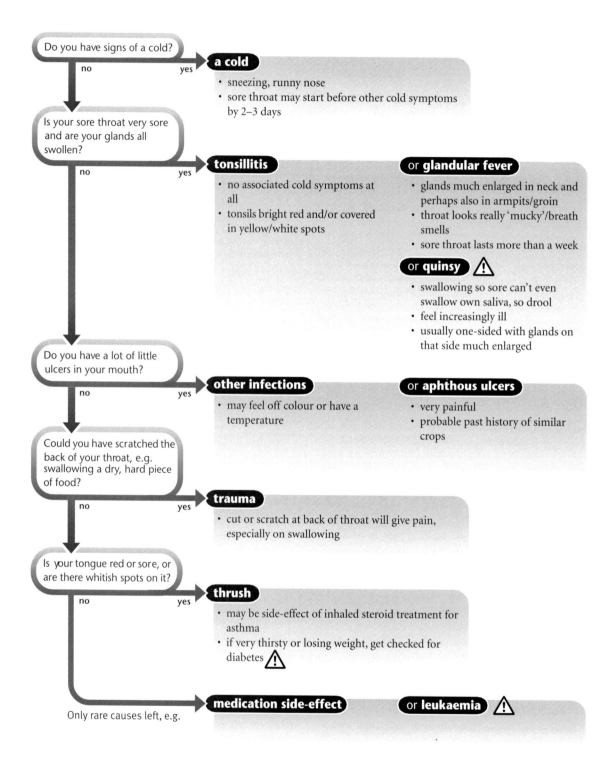

Do you have signs of a cold?   no   yes

a cold
- sneezing, runny nose
- sore throat may start before other cold symptoms by 2–3 days

Is your sore throat very sore and are your glands all swollen?   no   yes

tonsillitis
- no associated cold symptoms at all
- tonsils bright red and/or covered in yellow/white spots

or glandular fever
- glands much enlarged in neck and perhaps also in armpits/groin
- throat looks really 'mucky'/breath smells
- sore throat lasts more than a week

or quinsy ⚠
- swallowing so sore can't even swallow own saliva, so drool
- feel increasingly ill
- usually one-sided with glands on that side much enlarged

Do you have a lot of little ulcers in your mouth?   no   yes

other infections
- may feel off colour or have a temperature

or aphthous ulcers
- very painful
- probable past history of similar crops

Could you have scratched the back of your throat, e.g. swallowing a dry, hard piece of food?   no   yes

trauma
- cut or scratch at back of throat will give pain, especially on swallowing

Is your tongue red or sore, or are there whitish spots on it?   no   yes

thrush
- may be side-effect of inhaled steroid treatment for asthma
- if very thirsty or losing weight, get checked for diabetes ⚠

Only rare causes left, e.g.

medication side-effect   **or leukaemia** ⚠

A cold Colds are infections caused by viruses which irritate the upper part of the airways – this includes the ears, nose, and throat.

Treatment There is no cure for a cold, so there's no point in seeing your GP. Antibiotics don't help at all. The symptoms settle on their own after a few days – your throat will be helped by soluble aspirin gargles or paracetamol, and plenty of fluids.

Tonsillitis The tonsils are two lumps of gristle which are part of the immune system and which sit in your throat, one on each side of the dangly bit (the 'uvula'). When infected by bacteria, they become swollen, painful, and either red like a strawberry or covered with pus.

Treatment Even the docs can't decide on this one. Some GPs will always give antibiotics, some don't prescribe them at all, but most make a judgement on each individual case. Research shows that, if antibiotics help, all they do is speed up recovery by a day or two. If the attack is mild and you feel reasonably well, try the self-help measures mentioned under 'A cold'. If your throat is very sore, you're feverish, and feeling terrible, then it's worth contacting your GP.

Glandular fever This is a type of virus, usually passed on by close contact. It causes symptoms very similar to tonsillitis. In some cases the throat can become very sore, causing difficulty in swallowing, and you might continue to feel out of sorts for some weeks after the soreness has disappeared.

Treatment Some doctors will arrange a blood test to confirm that you have glandular fever. This isn't always necessary, though – your GP may make the diagnosis just by looking at your throat, and point out that it's simply a virus which lasts a bit longer than most. Or you may have such a mild attack that you don't bother to see your GP at all. Besides, there's no specific treatment for this problem other than the simple measures outlined above. So knowing you've got glandular fever doesn't help much, apart from providing an explanation as to why your throat might feel sore – or you feel lousy – for longer than usual. The rare case which makes it impossible to swallow and makes you feel dreadful does need medical attention, of course.

Trauma A swallowed bone or badly chewed food – especially chips or crisps – can scratch the back of the throat, causing an area of soreness.

Treatment Just take painkillers if necessary, drink plenty of fluids, and chew your food carefully so as not to aggravate it – it'll heal in a few days.

Quinsy This is an abscess around one tonsil – an unusual complication of tonsillitis.

Treatment See your GP. An early one may be cured by antibiotics. But if the abscess is fully developed, you'll need to go to hospital to have it lanced under anaesthetic.

Other infections There are a number of other germs – mainly viruses – which can cause a sore throat. Often, they produce lots of small, painful ulcers which can also appear on the lips, gums, and tongue.

Treatment All that's usually needed is the standard treatment of aspirin gargles or paracetamol and plenty of cool fluids. It's only worth seeing your GP if it's making you feel very ill or you're having trouble swallowing any fluids because of the pain.

Thrush This is a fungus infection. Most women know about it causing itching and discharge when it infects the vagina – but it can affect the throat too, in either sex.

Treatment Get some anti-fungal lozenges or medicine from your GP. This problem is unusual in the under 45s – the likeliest cause in this age group is a side-effect of asthma inhalers. Steroid inhalers tend to encourage the thrush fungus to grow in the throat. If you have asthma and you use this type of treatment, try to improve your inhaler technique (check the patient leaflet supplied with the inhaler) and gargle some water after each dose. Your GP may prescribe a 'spacer' – a gizmo which attaches to your inhaler and directs the spray into your lungs rather than the back of your throat. Rarely, in people not on asthma inhalers, thrush infection of the throat may be a sign of diabetes or an immune problem – your GP may check out these possibilities.

Aphthous ulcers These are explained in the 'Mouth ulcers' section (p.98). As they can occur anywhere in the mouth, they are sometimes the cause of a sore patch in the throat.

Treatment There is no cure, but you can try various gels and pastes from the chemist which, if used early, can help clear up an attack – but it can be tricky applying it to the throat as it'll tend to make you gag.

Medical rarities There are some rare medical problems which can cause a persistent and severe sore throat – these include serious blood disorders and the side-effects of some treatments (such as some anti-thyroid or anti-epilepsy drugs).

Treatment If you think you fit into this category, which is highly unlikely, see your GP to get the problem checked out.

Stiff or painful neck

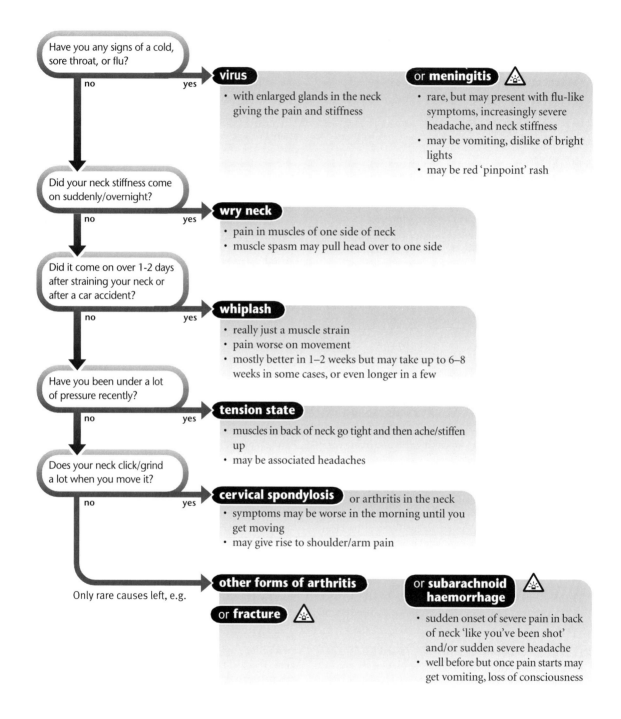

Have you any signs of a cold, sore throat, or flu?

no → yes →

virus
- with enlarged glands in the neck giving the pain and stiffness

or **meningitis**
- rare, but may present with flu-like symptoms, increasingly severe headache, and neck stiffness
- may be vomiting, dislike of bright lights
- may be red 'pinpoint' rash

Did your neck stiffness come on suddenly/overnight?

no → yes →

wry neck
- pain in muscles of one side of neck
- muscle spasm may pull head over to one side

Did it come on over 1-2 days after straining your neck or after a car accident?

no → yes →

whiplash
- really just a muscle strain
- pain worse on movement
- mostly better in 1–2 weeks but may take up to 6–8 weeks in some cases, or even longer in a few

Have you been under a lot of pressure recently?

no → yes →

tension state
- muscles in back of neck go tight and then ache/stiffen up
- may be associated headaches

Does your neck click/grind a lot when you move it?

no → yes →

cervical spondylosis or arthritis in the neck
- symptoms may be worse in the morning until you get moving
- may give rise to shoulder/arm pain

Only rare causes left, e.g.

other forms of arthritis

or **fracture**

or **subarachnoid haemorrhage**
- sudden onset of severe pain in back of neck 'like you've been shot' and/or sudden severe headache
- well before but once pain starts may get vomiting, loss of consciousness

If you get a sudden severe pain in the back of your neck or increasing headache and neck stiffness, seek medical help immediately to exclude subarachnoid haemorrhage or meningitis.

Stiff or painful neck

Virus with enlarged glands in the neck When you have a virus causing a sore throat or flu, the glands in your neck may swell. This is a sign that your body's immune system is fighting off the germ. The enlarged glands can irritate the neck muscles, resulting in stiffness.

Treatment You're unlikely to need much more than some paracetamol or aspirin, plenty of fluids, and some sympathy.

Wry neck This is spasm of the neck muscles. It may be caused by a trapped nerve in the neck or by sleeping in an awkward position. The muscles cramp up, causing pain, stiffness, and sometimes pulling your head over to one side.

Treatment Try heat, massage, and painkillers from the chemist, and get the neck moving as quickly as possible. The problem usually sorts itself out within a couple of days. A rare type, called 'spasmodic torticollis', keeps coming back and occasionally needs specialized treatment – so see your GP if you get repeated attacks of wry neck.

Tension state If you are uptight, your muscles tend to tense up – particularly in the neck. This causes a constant dull ache and stiffness.

Treatment Massage, heat, and neck exercises usually work well; you can use over-the-counter painkillers if necessary too. Also, try to get to the root of the problem – either by sorting out whatever it is in your life that's getting you tense, or by winding down more. Getting fitter and trying relaxation exercises will help. For further details, see the 'Feeling tense' section (p. 64).

Whiplash This results from a sudden stretching of the neck muscles. They become inflamed, leading to pain and stiffness which often doesn't appear until a day or so after the injury. A typical cause is a car accident in which you are shunted in the rear: your head suddenly jerks back, then forwards, like the 'crack' of a whip.

Treatment The key thing is to get your neck moving as quickly as possible. As it may be very stiff and painful, you may need regular and strongish painkillers – ask your pharmacist for advice. As with most stiff necks, massage and heat will also help. Many people find wearing a soft collar effective, but be warned: research shows that if the collar is worn for more than a couple of days, the stiffness takes longer to settle. So if you have been given a collar, get rid of it as soon as possible, grit your teeth, and exercise that neck. While most whiplash injuries get better quickly, a few take months, or even longer, to heal. X-rays don't help at all, and other treatments like physiotherapy usually make very little difference.

Cervical spondylosis The spine, including the neck, is made up of a column of small bones which interlock with each other via lots of very small joints. As you get older, these joints suffer wear and tear (osteoarthritis). In the neck, this is known as cervical spondylosis. It can result in a clicking, grinding neck with attacks of pain and stiffness.

Treatment All the treatments already mentioned will also help this problem. Again, neck exercise is important to relieve stiffness. Anti-inflammatory drugs such as ibuprofen (available from the chemist) can be very effective. Cervical spondylosis is sometimes worse in the morning, probably because you accidentally twist your neck into uncomfortable positions during the night. A butterfly pillow – a specially shaped headrest which can easily be made by tying some string tightly around the middle of a pillow so that it forms a 'bow tie' shape – can help by keeping your head still at night.

Other forms of arthritis Special types of arthritis, such as rheumatoid arthritis, which affect various joints and, sometimes, other parts of the body too – can cause trouble in the neck.

Treatment Your GP will probably try you on anti-inflammatory drugs, but you are also likely to be referred to a rheumatologist (joint specialist) for further treatment..

Fracture A severe injury, such as diving into shallow water and bashing your head on the bottom of the pool, can break one of the small bones in the neck. Not surprisingly, this will cause severe pain and neck spasm.

Treatment You are unlikely to have to worry about self-treatment too much – chances are, you're already in hospital.

Meningitis This is an inflammation of the lining of the brain. One of its effects is to send the neck muscles into spasm, so it's difficult to flex your head – in other words, to get your chin on to your chest. It's serious, but rare, and if you're unfortunate enough to be suffering from meningitis, you're likely to be complaining of rather more than a stiff neck.

Treatment Straight to hospital without delay.

Subarachnoid haemorrhage This is explained in the 'Headache' section (p. 70). Like meningitis, it inflames the brain lining, causing a stiff neck.

Swelling on/around the face

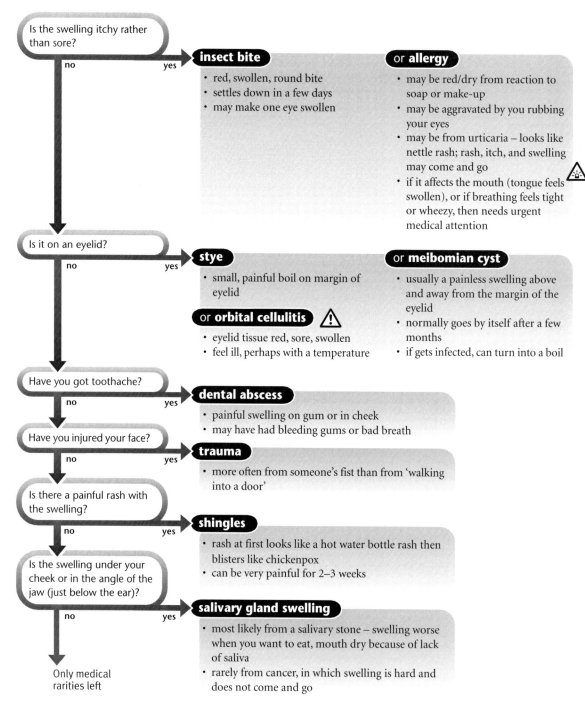

Is the swelling itchy rather than sore?
no / yes

insect bite
- red, swollen, round bite
- settles down in a few days
- may make one eye swollen

or **allergy**
- may be red/dry from reaction to soap or make-up
- may be aggravated by you rubbing your eyes
- may be from urticaria – looks like nettle rash; rash, itch, and swelling may come and go
- if it affects the mouth (tongue feels swollen), or if breathing feels tight or wheezy, then needs urgent medical attention

Is it on an eyelid?
no / yes

stye
- small, painful boil on margin of eyelid

or **orbital cellulitis**
- eyelid tissue red, sore, swollen
- feel ill, perhaps with a temperature

or **meibomian cyst**
- usually a painless swelling above and away from the margin of the eyelid
- normally goes by itself after a few months
- if gets infected, can turn into a boil

Have you got toothache?
no / yes

dental abscess
- painful swelling on gum or in cheek
- may have had bleeding gums or bad breath

Have you injured your face?
no / yes

trauma
- more often from someone's fist than from 'walking into a door'

Is there a painful rash with the swelling?
no / yes

shingles
- rash at first looks like a hot water bottle rash then blisters like chickenpox
- can be very painful for 2–3 weeks

Is the swelling under your cheek or in the angle of the jaw (just below the ear)?
no / yes

salivary gland swelling
- most likely from a salivary stone – swelling worse when you want to eat, mouth dry because of lack of saliva
- rarely from cancer, in which swelling is hard and does not come and go

Only medical rarities left

If an allergic rash/swelling on the face makes your tongue feel swollen, or if your breathing feels tight/wheezy, seek medical attention urgently.

Insect bite Because the skin around the eye is quite slack, it can swell impressively after an insect bite.

Treatment It'll go on its own after a day or so. An ice-pack or antihistamine tablets (like you'd use for hay fever – available from the chemist) will help.

Stye This is an infection of the eyelid – the germ gets in around an eyelash, making the lid swollen and painful.

Treatment It'll sort itself out in a few days. Plucking out the eyelash in the centre of the stye may help. If the whole eye is getting red and sticky, you're probably developing conjunctivitis – try gently bathing the eye for a couple of days, but if it persists, see your GP for some antibiotic ointment.

Meibomian cyst If one of the tiny glands in your eyelid ('meibomian' glands) gets blocked, you end up with a pea-sized lump. This is common and harmless.

Treatment This can be left alone – it may eventually disappear on its own. If it doesn't and it's a nuisance, it can be cured with a very small operation: your GP can arrange this for you by referring you to an ophthalmologist (eye specialist).

Trauma You don't have to be a rocket scientist to work out that a bash in the face might cause swelling.

Treatment If you've had a significant bump – say a punch or an elbow in the face – causing swelling, you need to go to casualty for an X-ray, as you may have a fracture.

Dental abscess This is an infection of the root of a tooth. The germ gets into the gum, making it swell.

Treatment You'll need some antibiotics and painkillers, so get to a dentist asap.

Allergy Two types of allergy can make your face swell. One is caused by something which has been in contact with your face, such as soap or shampoo. This tends to make the skin swell slightly and get itchy or sore, and is known as 'allergic contact eczema'. The other (called 'angio-oedema') results from a severe allergy to something which gets into your system. It has various causes, including foods, medications, and insects bites or stings – the reaction can be quite severe, so that your lips, tongue, or even your throat swell. In both types, you may previously have had no problems with whatever it is you've now developed an allergy to – it doesn't have to be something which is completely 'new' to you.

Treatment Treat allergic contact eczema with hydrocortisone 1% cream (available over the counter) and by avoiding whatever has caused it. Angio-oedema can get quite nasty, so you'll need to see your GP urgently for advice and treatment. Very rarely, the swelling can block your windpipe, so if you're having difficulty breathing, you need to go straight to hospital. Once you've been sorted out, you need to look at ways of preventing future attacks. Try to figure out what caused it, and be careful as far as possible to steer well clear of what you're allergic to in the future. Keep some antihistamines handy (available from the chemist) to use at the first sign of any trouble – they may nip another attack in the bud. If it turns out you've got a really severe allergy – to nuts or wasp stings for example – you may be given adrenaline (in the form of an injection) to use in case of future problems. Make sure you, and your nearest and dearest, know how to use it.

Shingles This is explained, and the treatment discussed, in the 'Blisters' section (p. 30). If it occurs on the face, it can cause swelling on one side, especially on or around the eyelid – even before the blisters of shingles appear.

Orbital cellulitis See the 'Red eye' section (p. 130).

Salivary gland swellings The salivary glands produce the saliva which lubricates food when you chew. They are found just below your ear (parotid glands) and under your jaw (submandibular glands). They can swell for a number of reasons, including infections (such as mumps, although this is unusual nowadays) and stones (gravelly bits which block the tubes carrying the saliva). Very rarely, a persistent swelling of the parotid gland is caused by a growth.

Treatment This depends on the cause. Many of the infections are caused by viruses and go away on their own. Other types may need antibiotics, so if the swelling is very sore, showing no signs of going down, or you feel ill or feverish, see your GP. Swellings caused by stones can be cured by stimulating the flow of saliva (with lemon drops, for example) or with a small operation. Growths need sorting out by a specialist.

Medical rarities A few small-print problems can make the face puff up (such as an underactive thyroid gland or the side-effects of steroid treatment) or cause an obviously swollen area (such as bone or sinus cancer).

Treatment These are very unlikely to be the cause of your problem. If you're concerned, discuss the situation with your GP.

Swollen glands

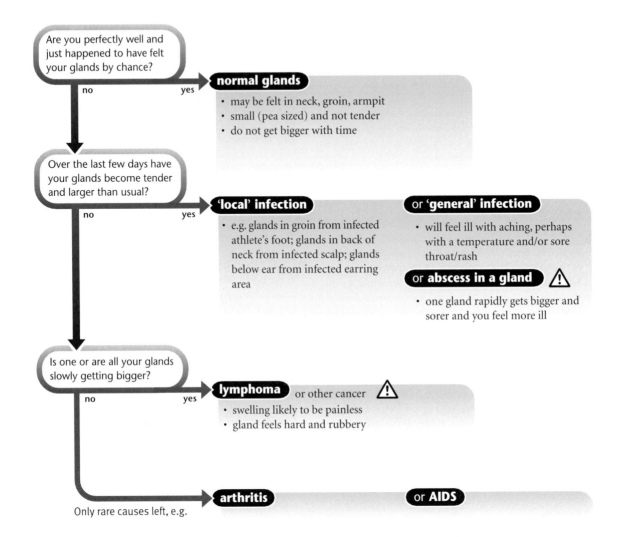

Are you perfectly well and just happened to have felt your glands by chance?

no / yes

normal glands
- may be felt in neck, groin, armpit
- small (pea sized) and not tender
- do not get bigger with time

Over the last few days have your glands become tender and larger than usual?

no / yes

'local' infection
- e.g. glands in groin from infected athlete's foot; glands in back of neck from infected scalp; glands below ear from infected earring area

or 'general' infection
- will feel ill with aching, perhaps with a temperature and/or sore throat/rash

or abscess in a gland ⚠
- one gland rapidly gets bigger and sorer and you feel more ill

Is one or are all your glands slowly getting bigger?

no / yes

lymphoma or other cancer ⚠
- swelling likely to be painless
- gland feels hard and rubbery

Only rare causes left, e.g.

arthritis   or **AIDS**

Remember: ⚠ means see your GP sharpish; ⚠ means an urgent hospital job

Normal glands Glands are found in various parts of the body – particularly the neck, the armpits, and the groin. They are a part of your immune system, which helps fight off infections. If you're slim, it's quite normal to be able to feel these glands as pea-sized, non-tender lumps which stay roughly the same size most of the time.

Treatment Being able to feel these glands is entirely normal, so no treatment is needed.

'Local' infection If a germ gets into one part of your body, the glands nearby will swell as they try to fight it off. For example, your neck glands will enlarge if you get a sore throat, and the glands in your groin may swell if you pick up a sexually transmitted germ.

Treatment The glands themselves don't need any treatment – the fact that they've swollen just means they're doing their job. But the infection which has made them swell may need sorting out. So unless it's just a case of your neck glands swelling up a bit with a mild sore throat, see your GP.

'General' infection Some germs don't stick in one area – instead they get right into your system, making all your glands swell up. Examples include viruses like glandular fever and German measles (rare nowadays, as almost all children are immunized against this).

Treatment Again, the glands themselves don't need treating. The fact that they've swollen means they're trying to fight off the germ. In fact, because most of these infections are caused by viruses, there's usually no magic cure – you simply have to wait for them to burn themselves out. Paracetamol will help the fever, aches and pains, and sore throat which often go with this type of problem; for more information on treating glandular fever, see the 'Sore throat' section (p. 136). If you feel very ill and feverish, you ought to discuss the situation with your GP.

Abscess in a gland If a particular type of germ gets into a gland, it can sometimes produce a large boil-like swelling, full of pus. This is an abscess.

Treatment If it's only just come on, antibiotics may cure it. But if it's developed into a full-blown abscess, it'll need lancing to let the pus out. Either way, you'll need to see your GP.

Lymphoma This is a cancer of the lymph glands.

Treatment It's unlikely that this is the cause of your problem, but if you're worried it could be, you obviously need to see your GP asap. If she shares your concern, she'll probably run some tests and refer you to a specialist. The treatment is unpleasant – chemotherapy (powerful drugs) or radiotherapy (radiation beam treatment) – but offers a chance of cure.

Other rare medical conditions Lots of other rarities can make the glands of the body swell. These include some types of arthritis, other cancers, AIDS, and the side-effects of some medication.

Treatment See your GP if you're worried that you might have one of these unusual causes. She'll arrange any necessary tests and treatment.

Tired all the time

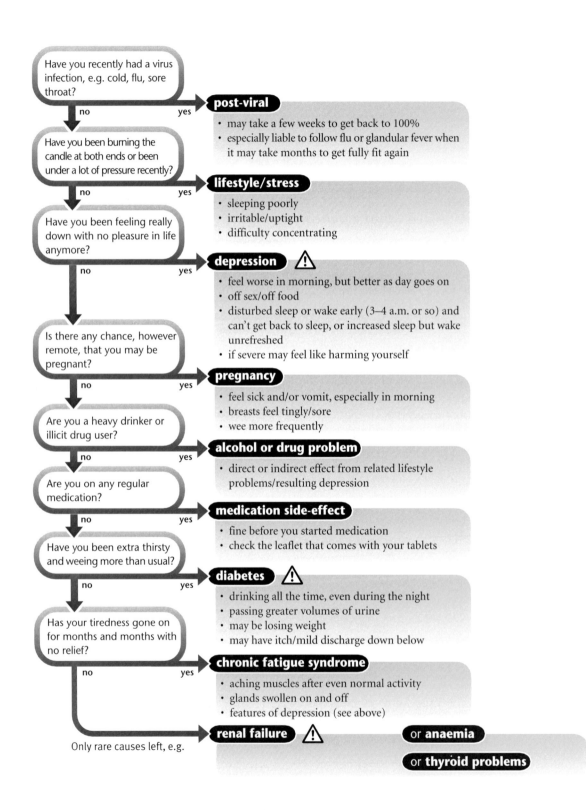

Have you recently had a virus infection, e.g. cold, flu, sore throat?

no · yes

post-viral
- may take a few weeks to get back to 100%
- especially liable to follow flu or glandular fever when it may take months to get fully fit again

Have you been burning the candle at both ends or been under a lot of pressure recently?

no · yes

lifestyle/stress
- sleeping poorly
- irritable/uptight
- difficulty concentrating

Have you been feeling really down with no pleasure in life anymore?

no · yes

depression ⚠
- feel worse in morning, but better as day goes on
- off sex/off food
- disturbed sleep or wake early (3–4 a.m. or so) and can't get back to sleep, or increased sleep but wake unrefreshed
- if severe may feel like harming yourself

Is there any chance, however remote, that you may be pregnant?

no · yes

pregnancy
- feel sick and/or vomit, especially in morning
- breasts feel tingly/sore
- wee more frequently

Are you a heavy drinker or illicit drug user?

no · yes

alcohol or drug problem
- direct or indirect effect from related lifestyle problems/resulting depression

Are you on any regular medication?

no · yes

medication side-effect
- fine before you started medication
- check the leaflet that comes with your tablets

Have you been extra thirsty and weeing more than usual?

no · yes

diabetes ⚠
- drinking all the time, even during the night
- passing greater volumes of urine
- may be losing weight
- may have itch/mild discharge down below

Has your tiredness gone on for months and months with no relief?

no · yes

chronic fatigue syndrome
- aching muscles after even normal activity
- glands swollen on and off
- features of depression (see above)

Only rare causes left, e.g.

renal failure ⚠   **or anaemia**

or thyroid problems

Lifestyle/stress Tiredness is one of the complaints your GP deals with daily. If there are no other particular symptoms, such as weight loss, it's very unlikely to be caused by a physical disease. Research has shown that, when questioned, up to a third of people feel 'tired all the time'. In most cases there isn't one specific cause – the tiredness is due to a mixture of things such as poor or irregular sleep, lack of physical exercise, and pressure at work. Stress usually plays a part: it's exhausting being uptight all the time.

Treatment There's no magic pill, so don't bother your chemist or doctor. A sensible approach is to take a long hard look at your lifestyle and make some constructive changes. It's important to sort out your sleeping habits: go to bed at a set time as far as possible and try to get more sleep, but avoid daytime naps and lying in. You'll sleep, and feel, better if you increase the amount of physical exercise you take. Try to sort out any sources of stress in your life and wind down with some relaxation therapy (see the 'Feeling tense' section, p. 64).

Post-viral Any recent virus – especially influenza and glandular fever – can leave you feeling below par for some weeks. This is particularly the case if your lifestyle isn't particularly restful or you've made a very quick return to work.

Treatment There is no specific treatment for this – you simply have to be patient and try some of the measures outlined above while you wait for your energy levels to return to normal.

Depression This is explained, and its treatment outlined, in the 'Feeling down' section (p. 62).

Pregnancy Tiredness is one of many symptoms which you might notice in early pregnancy.

Treatment This is usually caused by the hormone changes rather than anaemia so iron pills are unlikely to help (and you'll be checked for anaemia with blood tests anyway).

Medication side-effect Some prescribed treatments, such as pills for blood pressure or antidepressants, can cause tiredness as a side-effect.

Treatment Check the leaflet in the treatment pack to see if tiredness is a side-effect. If it is, then speak to your GP. It can be difficult to know whether or not to blame the treatment as tiredness is so common anyway. If your GP thinks your medication could be the cause, then she may be able to stop it or switch you to an alternative.

Alcohol or drug problem Alcohol or drugs can cause tiredness in a number of ways. They can directly sap energy levels; they can make your life chaotic, resulting in a poor diet, no exercise, and a lack of sleep; and they can cause depression.

Treatment Cut down – or better still, stop – the substance abuse and get a grip on your lifestyle. If you find it difficult and want help, check out your local drug or alcohol services or see your GP.

Diabetes If your body fails to produce enough of the chemical 'insulin', your blood sugar starts to rise: this is diabetes. It's quite common, affecting two in every 100 people, but no one knows exactly why it happens. The high sugar level in your blood can cause a number of problems, including tiredness.

Treatment See your doc asap – and take a specimen of wee with you, as she'll want to test this. If it does turn out that you have diabetes, you'll need a special diet, probably with either tablets or insulin injections.

Chronic fatigue syndrome This is known by a variety of other names – in the past, 'yuppy flu' and, more recently, 'ME' (myalgic encephalomyelitis). Chronic fatigue syndrome (CFS), meaning 'long-term tiredness', is a better name, but this is where the agreement ends and the controversy begins as there's still a lot of debate about what CFS is exactly and what causes it. Some heated arguments have raged about whether the problem is in the mind or body, but most doctors now agree it's probably a bit of both. CFS is a feeling of severe tiredness which won't go away and which may be linked with aching muscles, swollen glands, and feelings of depression. No one is sure what triggers it – it may be a virus, an emotional upset, or something else. Nor does anyone know what keeps it going, although psychological factors are thought to play a part. These might include a negative or pessimistic attitude, an incorrect belief that 'a virus' is still lurking in the body, and an unwillingness to try even small amounts of exercise. In the worst cases, people can become very disabled and the symptoms can go on for years.

Treatment As no one can agree on what causes CFS, it's no surprise that the treatment depends very much on who you listen to. There is certainly no magic pill to sort out the problem. Doctors who've done a lot of research into CFS believe it's very important to take a positive approach and to avoid looking for miracle cures Gentle exercise, gradually increased, is likely to help. It's important not to overdo it at first, otherwise the resulting exhaustion will make you want to 'give up', so you'll be one step forwards and two back, and prone to developing a 'can't do' attitude. Antidepressants help some patients if feeling down is a big part of the problem. Your best bet is to discuss the situation with your GP.

Other medical problems Tiredness can be a feature of many medical problems such as anaemia, thyroid trouble, and kidney failure. It's pretty unlikely you'll have any of these.

Treatment See your GP, who'll arrange the necessary tests if she's concerned.

Tremor

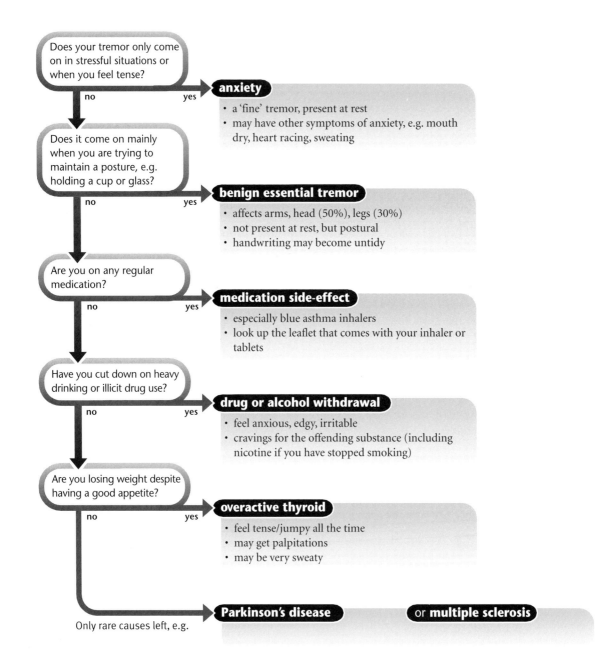

Anxiety If you're frightened or angry, you'll know it's normal to tremble. This can happen constantly if you're feeling very tense all the time, or occasionally, if you get really anxious in certain situations.

Treatment The treatment of anxiety is discussed in the 'Palpitations' (p. 116) and 'Feeling tense' (p. 64) sections – exactly the same principles apply with tremor. If the tremor is a real problem – particularly if it affects your performance when you get uptight doing, for example, a speech or a presentation – your GP may be able to give you some tablets to ease it.

Benign essential tremor Everyone experiences a tremor, but most aren't aware of it because it's very slight (you can prove this by putting a piece of A4 paper over your outstretched hand – you'll see the edges of the paper shake). In some people, for some reason, this normal tremor is much more obvious – this is called benign essential tremor. It often runs in families.

Treatment This is harmless and will not develop into anything more serious, so it's safe to leave it alone. You'll probably find that a small alcoholic drink gets rid of the problem completely for a short period of time, though for obvious reasons this can't be recommended as a regular treatment. If the tremor is a real nuisance, discuss it with your GP. She might prescribe some tablets which can help ease the problem.

Medication side-effect Some prescribed treatments, such as drugs for severe psychiatric conditions, can cause tremor as a side-effect. It can also be caused by certain asthma inhalers (the 'treater' inhalers, such as salbutamol and terbutaline), especially if you're using them too much.

Treatment If you think your medication might be causing a tremor, discuss the situation with your GP. When the tremor is caused by overuse of asthma inhalers, you obviously need to ease up on them and you may need to see your GP – using too many inhalers probably means that your asthma isn't under proper control, so the doc may want to alter your treatment. Of course, if you've been bashing the inhalers because you're having a bad asthma attack, you need to see your GP urgently.

Drug or alcohol withdrawal If your body has been used to regular doses of a drug or alcohol which is suddenly stopped, you may suffer a 'withdrawal syndrome' – symptoms caused by the body craving the drug. Most people are familiar with this happening with illegal addictive drugs, but it can also be caused by suddenly stopping alcohol and some prescribed treatments. A tremor is one of the signs of drug withdrawal.

Treatment If the tremor isn't too bad, and other symptoms of withdrawal aren't a great problem, then just sit it out – it'll settle down in due course. But if the withdrawal syndrome is giving you real problems, seek help via your GP or the local drug or alcohol unit. You'll probably be given some medication as a 'substitute' for whatever your body is craving, and then weaned off this treatment slowly so you don't suffer bad withdrawal effects.

Overactive thyroid This is explained, and its treatment outlined, in the 'Excess sweating' section (p. 58).

Rare medical causes Diseases of the nervous system (such as Parkinson's disease or multiple sclerosis) can cause a tremor. But they're either very rare in women under 50, or are likely to be causing other, more worrying, symptoms than tremor and so are very unlikely to be the cause.

Treatment See your GP. If she shares your concerns, she'll refer you to a neurologist (nervous system specialist) for further tests.

Vaginal discharge

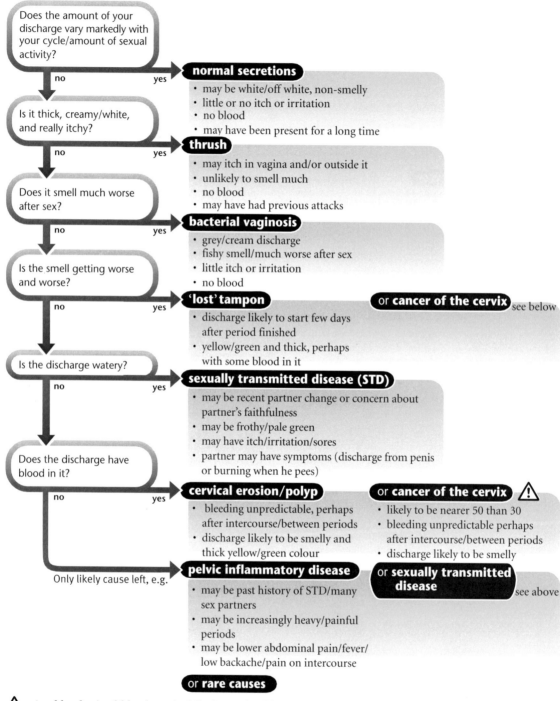

Does the amount of your discharge vary markedly with your cycle/amount of sexual activity?

no → yes →

normal secretions
- may be white/off white, non-smelly
- little or no itch or irritation
- no blood
- may have been present for a long time

Is it thick, creamy/white, and really itchy?

no → yes →

thrush
- may itch in vagina and/or outside it
- unlikely to smell much
- no blood
- may have had previous attacks

Does it smell much worse after sex?

no → yes →

bacterial vaginosis
- grey/cream discharge
- fishy smell/much worse after sex
- little itch or irritation
- no blood

Is the smell getting worse and worse?

no → yes →

'lost' tampon   **or cancer of the cervix** see below
- discharge likely to start few days after period finished
- yellow/green and thick, perhaps with some blood in it

Is the discharge watery?

no → yes →

sexually transmitted disease (STD)
- may be recent partner change or concern about partner's faithfulness
- may be frothy/pale green
- may have itch/irritation/sores
- partner may have symptoms (discharge from penis or burning when he pees)

Does the discharge have blood in it?

no → yes →

cervical erosion/polyp   **or cancer of the cervix** ⚠
- bleeding unpredictable, perhaps after intercourse/between periods
- discharge likely to be smelly and thick yellow/green colour

- likely to be nearer 50 than 30
- bleeding unpredictable perhaps after intercourse/between periods
- discharge likely to be smelly

Only likely cause left, e.g.

pelvic inflammatory disease   **or sexually transmitted disease** see above
- may be past history of STD/many sex partners
- may be increasingly heavy/painful periods
- may be lower abdominal pain/fever/low backache/pain on intercourse

or rare causes

 Any bloodstained/bloody vaginal discharge should be checked out by your doc to exclude cancer.

Vaginal discharge

Normal secretions Glands in the vagina produce a lubricating fluid which can sometimes appear as a discharge. Different women produce different amounts, and the quantity also varies with your cycle; it may be increased by pregnancy, the Pill, and the coil. A really stimulating sex life (first boyfriend or a new partner, for example) is another common cause. As this type of discharge is totally normal, it requires no treatment.

Thrush This is explained, and the treatment outlined, in the 'Vulval irritation and/or sores' section (p. 158).

Bacterial vaginosis No matter how hygienic you are, your vagina will play host to a number of germs – it's quite normal for them to live there, they usually cause no problems, and they're not passed on through sex. If there's a shift in the balance of the germ population, some of the bugs become more numerous and can then cause a discharge – this is bacterial vaginosis.

Treatment See your GP for a course of antibiotics. As it's not passed on sexually, there's no need to get your partner treated. Don't overdo the washing, thinking that you're not clean – by washing away some of the other germs, you allow the bacterial vaginosis bugs to multiply, making matters worse.

Sexually transmitted disease A variety of germs can be passed on through sex: trichomonas, gonorrhoea, chlamydia, and herpes. All may result in a discharge.

Treatment If you think you have a sexually transmitted infection, your best bet is to go to a local clinic for genito-urinary medicine (or 'special clinic'). You'll get the necessary treatment there and you'll also be checked for any other infections. Most hospitals have these clinics – just ring up and find out when you can be seen. It's worth getting your partner checked and treated too, otherwise you may get reinfected. For further information on herpes, see the 'Vulval irritation and/or sores' section (p. 158).

Cervical erosion or polyp These are explained, and the treatment outlined, in the 'Cervical erosion/polyp/cervicitis' part of the 'Abnormal or irregular vaginal bleeding' section (p. 16).

'Lost' tampon A forgotten tampon will produce a foul discharge.

Treatment Fish it out yourself if you can, otherwise your GP or practice nurse will oblige. If it's been there a while, or the discharge is particularly unpleasant, you may need a course of antibiotics – discuss the situation with your GP. Get the tampon removed as soon as possible as there is the small possibility of developing the serious condition 'toxic shock syndrome', in which infection gets into your bloodstream, making you very ill indeed.

Pelvic inflammatory disease This is explained, and the treatment outlined, in the 'Lower abdominal pain – recurrent' (p. 94) and 'Lower abdominal pain – one-off' (p. 92) sections.

Cancer of the cervix and other rare causes
Some cancers (such as cancer of the cervix, vagina, or womb) and ectopic pregnancy can announce themselves with a vaginal discharge.

Treatment These problems are unlikely to be the cause of your symptoms. If you're concerned, see your GP soon (urgently if you think you might have an ectopic pregnancy – see the 'Lower abdominal pain – one-off' section, p. 92), who will check the symptom out properly for you and, if necessary, refer you to a gynaecologist.

Vision problems

(If you have a red eye, see p. 130)

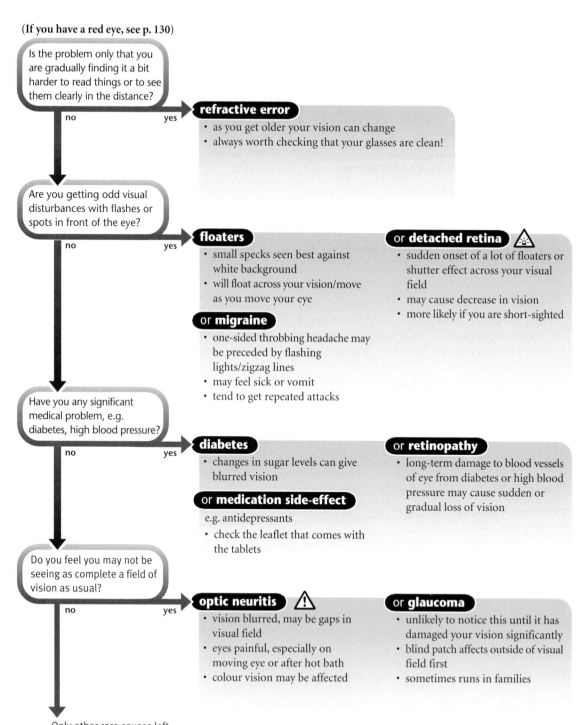

Is the problem only that you are gradually finding it a bit harder to read things or to see them clearly in the distance?

no → yes →

refractive error
- as you get older your vision can change
- always worth checking that your glasses are clean!

Are you getting odd visual disturbances with flashes or spots in front of the eye?

no → yes →

floaters
- small specks seen best against white background
- will float across your vision/move as you move your eye

or migraine
- one-sided throbbing headache may be preceded by flashing lights/zigzag lines
- may feel sick or vomit
- tend to get repeated attacks

or detached retina
- sudden onset of a lot of floaters or shutter effect across your visual field
- may cause decrease in vision
- more likely if you are short-sighted

Have you any significant medical problem, e.g. diabetes, high blood pressure?

no → yes →

diabetes
- changes in sugar levels can give blurred vision

or medication side-effect
e.g. antidepressants
- check the leaflet that comes with the tablets

or retinopathy
- long-term damage to blood vessels of eye from diabetes or high blood pressure may cause sudden or gradual loss of vision

Do you feel you may not be seeing as complete a field of vision as usual?

no → yes →

optic neuritis
- vision blurred, may be gaps in visual field
- eyes painful, especially on moving eye or after hot bath
- colour vision may be affected

or glaucoma
- unlikely to notice this until it has damaged your vision significantly
- blind patch affects outside of visual field first
- sometimes runs in families

Only other rare causes left

If you get a sudden onset of flashers/floaters, especially with decreased vision, or if you get a sudden loss of all or part of your field vision, seek medical attention urgently.

Refractive errors The eye is like a camera. The iris (the coloured part of your eye) is the aperture, letting the light in. It's focused by the lens and the cornea (the clear part of the front of the eye) on to the retina at the back of the eye – the equivalent of the film. Problems with the cornea, lens, or shape of the eye which stop the light from focusing on the retina properly are called 'refractive errors'. These include: short-sightedness, when you can see clearly close up but not in the distance; long-sightedness, when the reverse applies; and astigmatism, when the cornea is uneven causing blurring for far and near vision.

Treatment You don't need to do anything about it if it doesn't bother you – but make sure your eyesight is still OK for you to drive. If you want to sort it out, see your optician, who will be able to arrange glasses or contact lenses for you. You can also consider surgery which alters the curve of your cornea and so improves your vision. But bear in mind that the results aren't always fantastic, there can be side-effects, and it's only available privately, so you're likely to have to fork out loads of money.

Floaters Bits of debris can collect together inside the eye. These float around in the fluid inside the eyeball and are seen – particularly against a white background – as small specks or spidery shadows.

Treatment These can be a nuisance but are harmless. There's no treatment and they're usually permanent, although you get used to them so they become less noticeable in time. Very occasionally they can be a sign of a 'detached retina' (see 'Other rare medical problems' below), in which case they come on suddenly in a 'shower', usually with blurred vision. This needs assessment by your doc urgently.

Migraine If you get migraine, your eyesight may be affected before the headache comes on. This is because migraine starts with a tightening up of blood vessels to your brain, which can result in the part dealing with your vision being starved of oxygen for a short while. This can cause blurring, flashing lights, or tunnel vision. For further information about migraine, see the 'Headache' section (p. 70).

Diabetes This is explained in the Tired all the time' section (p.144). The high blood sugar in your bloodstream can lead to your vision blurring. Diabetes can also cause 'retinopathy' (see below).

Treatment See the 'Tired all the time' section (p. 144). If you're a 'known' diabetic, keep a close eye on your sugar readings and adjust your treatment if necessary and you're confident you know what to do – if not, contact your GP or the local diabetes nurse.

Retinopathy This means a disease of the retina. The commonest causes are high blood pressure and diabetes. They may cause more dramatic problems with vision such as sudden complete or partial blindness, but they may also result in gradual blurring.

Treatment See your GP to get the cause diagnosed and treated. This problem is sometimes picked up by your optician, who will then send you on to your doctor.

Medication side-effect Some prescribed medications, such as antidepressants, can affect the way your eye focuses, leading to blurred vision.

Treatment The problem will often correct itself as your body gets used to the treatment, so persevere for a while if you can. If it doesn't, speak to your GP – she may be able to stop the medication or swap it for something else.

Optic neuritis This is an inflammation of the nerve which supplies the retina. Some attacks are thought to be caused by a virus. Others are a part of – or the first sign of – multiple sclerosis (explained further in the 'Pins and needles and numbness' section, p. 118).

Treatment See your GP asap. If you're known to have multiple sclerosis, she may let the problem settle on its own or she may prescribe you steroid tablets. Otherwise, she'll probably just keep an eye on the situation as most attacks – especially those caused by viruses – go away on their own, although you may be left with some slight blurring or dimming of your vision (especially for colours). But if your doctor suspects you might be developing multiple sclerosis, she'll refer you to a neurologist (nerve specialist).

Glaucoma If the pressure of the fluid in your eye is too high, it can damage the retina. This problem sometimes runs in families. You're unlikely to notice it, especially at first, because it tends to affect only how well you see out of the corners of your eyes. It's more likely to be spotted during a routine check by your optician.

Treatment Your optician will give you a letter to take to your GP, who will then probably refer you to an eye specialist for a thorough check and, if necessary, treatment. If you have a family history of glaucoma but don't have any problem yourself, it's important to get regular eye checks from your optician.

Other rare medical problems A variety of small-print problems can blur your vision, including a detached retina, rare infections, and brain tumours.

Treatment It's highly unlikely you'll have any of these problems. If you're concerned, speak to your GP.

Vomiting

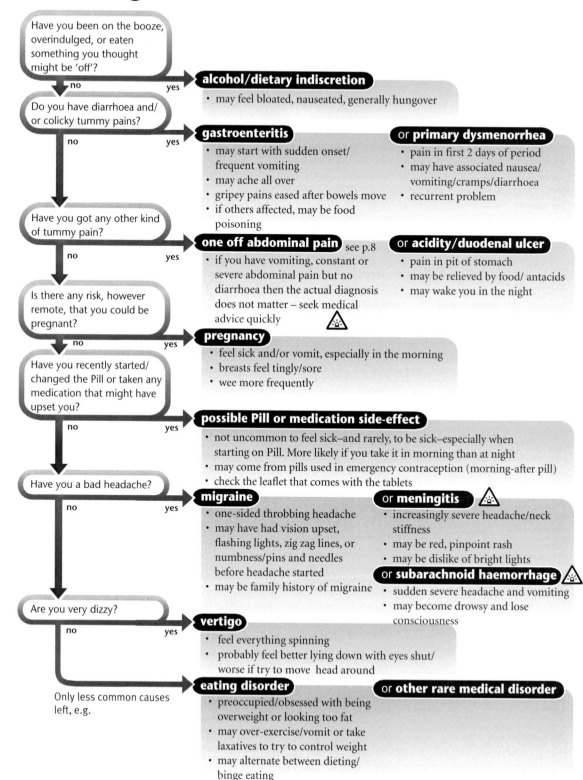

Have you been on the booze, overindulged, or eaten something you thought might be 'off'?

no / **yes**

alcohol/dietary indiscretion
- may feel bloated, nauseated, generally hungover

Do you have diarrhoea and/or colicky tummy pains?

no / **yes**

gastroenteritis
- may start with sudden onset/ frequent vomiting
- may ache all over
- gripey pains eased after bowels move
- if others affected, may be food poisoning

or primary dysmenorrhea
- pain in first 2 days of period
- may have associated nausea/ vomiting/cramps/diarrhoea
- recurrent problem

Have you got any other kind of tummy pain?

no / **yes**

one off abdominal pain see p.8
- if you have vomiting, constant or severe abdominal pain but no diarrhoea then the actual diagnosis does not matter – seek medical advice quickly

or acidity/duodenal ulcer
- pain in pit of stomach
- may be relieved by food/ antacids
- may wake you in the night

Is there any risk, however remote, that you could be pregnant?

no / **yes**

pregnancy
- feel sick and/or vomit, especially in the morning
- breasts feel tingly/sore
- wee more frequently

Have you recently started/ changed the Pill or taken any medication that might have upset you?

no / **yes**

possible Pill or medication side-effect
- not uncommon to feel sick–and rarely, to be sick–especially when starting on Pill. More likely if you take it in morning than at night
- may come from pills used in emergency contraception (morning-after pill)
- check the leaflet that comes with the tablets

Have you a bad headache?

no / **yes**

migraine
- one-sided throbbing headache
- may have had vision upset, flashing lights, zig zag lines, or numbness/pins and needles before headache started
- may be family history of migraine

or meningitis
- increasingly severe headache/neck stiffness
- may be red, pinpoint rash
- may be dislike of bright lights

or subarachnoid haemorrhage
- sudden severe headache and vomiting
- may become drowsy and lose consciousness

Are you very dizzy?

no / **yes**

vertigo
- feel everything spinning
- probably feel better lying down with eyes shut/ worse if try to move head around

Only less common causes left, e.g.

eating disorder
- preoccupied/obsessed with being overweight or looking too fat
- may over-exercise/vomit or take laxatives to try to control weight
- may alternate between dieting/ binge eating

or other rare medical disorder

If you have vomiting with sudden severe headache/pain in the back of your neck, or increasing headache and neck stiffness, seek medical help immediately to exclude subarachnoid haemorrhage or meningitis.

If you have vomiting with abdominal pain (not gripey with diarrhoea) then there may be a serious cause and you must seek medical advice immediately.

Alcohol/dietary indiscretion Vomiting after, say a garlic-soaked meal and a few bottles of wine is your body's way of saying 'thanks, but no thanks'.

Treatment This is an unpleasant but perfectly normal reaction, and so needs no specific treatment. You may want to treat the hangover the following morning, though: plenty of non-alcoholic fluids, painkillers for the headache, and antacids for any belly ache. And as regards prevention – it's simply a case of being more restrained in future.

Gastroenteritis This is explained, and the treatment outlined, in the 'Abdominal pain – one-off' section (p. 8).

One-off abdominal pain Many causes of severe abdominal pain produce vomiting, including appendicitis, ulcers, renal colic, gallstones, pancreatitis, and bowel obstruction. For more details, see the 'Abdominal pain – one-off' section (p. 8).

Medication side-effect Lots of different medications can irritate the stomach, leading to vomiting. Examples include anti-inflammatory drugs (such as ibuprofen) and antibiotics. Powerful drugs for cancers (known as 'chemotherapy') can cause severe vomiting, but if you're unlucky enough to be on this type of treatment, you'll have been warned about this side-effect – and you'll probably have been prescribed something to counteract it. It's very rare for the Pill to cause vomiting, but it can be a problem with the morning-after pill.

Treatment If the offending treatment was prescribed by your doc, discuss the situation with her. But if you bought the treatment over the counter, either simply stop it or have a word with your chemist. If you're sick within three hours of taking the morning-after pill, you need to seek medical advice because if it's not getting into your system, it may not work.

Migraine This is explained, and the treatment outlined, in the 'Headache' section (p. 70).

Pregnancy Nausea and vomiting, especially in the morning, are well-known early signs of pregnancy and are caused by the changes in your hormones. Later in pregnancy, the same symptoms may be caused by acid in the gullet ('reflux oesophagitis').

Treatment If it happens at all, this problem usually comes on in the early stages of pregnancy, settling down after the first three months. Having some dry biscuits or toast in bed before getting up, and avoiding fatty foods, can ease the symptoms while you wait for them to go. But if you're having terrible trouble with sickness, or you feel unwell with it, see your GP – she may be able to provide you with anti-sickness pills or, if you're getting dehydrated, she'll send you to hospital to have fluids through a drip. Vomiting caused by acid in the gullet can be treated with a liquid antacid from the chemist (if you're unsure whether it's OK to take when you're pregnant, check with the pharmacist or your GP); some of the tips explained in the 'Reflux oesophagitis' part of the 'Indigestion' section (p. 78) will help too.

Vertigo Many causes of vertigo (a feeling of unsteadiness or of the world spinning around) can lead to vomiting. The problem is explained fully, and treatment discussed, in the 'Dizziness' section (p. 52).

Eating disorder This is explained and the treatment discussed, in the 'Weight loss' section (p. 164). Vomiting is usually 'self-induced' – a finger down the throat job.

Primary dysmenorrhoea This is the medical term for 'normal' period pains, which can sometimes be so severe as to cause vomiting. For further details, see the 'Painful periods' section (p. 116).

Acidity/duodenal ulcer This can show itself with a 'bang', causing severe stomach pain, or it can grumble off and on for some time – more details, and advice about treatment, are given in the 'Abdominal pain – one-off' section (p. 8). Bad bouts can inflame the stomach lining so badly that you end up with repeated bouts of vomiting.

Rare and serious medical problems There are huge numbers of pretty nasty medical conditions which can cause vomiting – but they usually come to light through other symptoms. They include meningitis, subarachnoid haemorrhage and brain tumours (see 'Headache' section, p. 70), kidney failure, and stomach cancer.

Treatment It's very unlikely that you'll have any of these problems. Meningitis and subarachnoid haemorrhage require the services of an urgent ambulance. For anything else, you need to see your GP asap.

Vomiting up blood

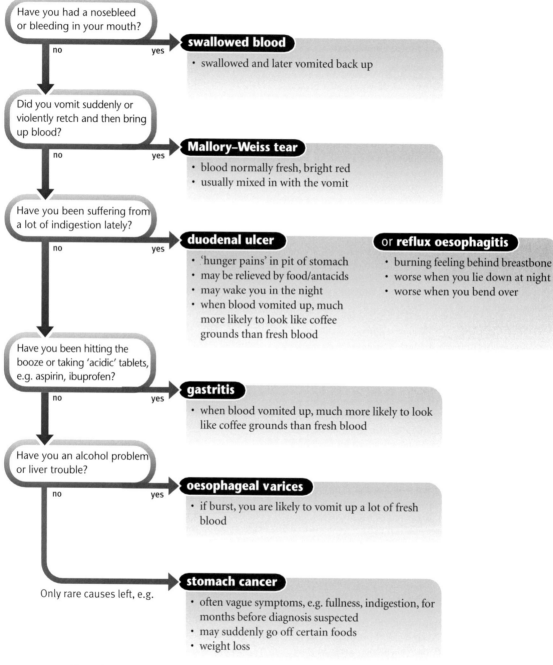

Have you had a nosebleed or bleeding in your mouth?
— no / yes →

swallowed blood
• swallowed and later vomited back up

Did you vomit suddenly or violently retch and then bring up blood?
— no / yes →

Mallory–Weiss tear
• blood normally fresh, bright red
• usually mixed in with the vomit

Have you been suffering from a lot of indigestion lately?
— no / yes →

duodenal ulcer
• 'hunger pains' in pit of stomach
• may be relieved by food/antacids
• may wake you in the night
• when blood vomited up, much more likely to look like coffee grounds than fresh blood

or reflux oesophagitis
• burning feeling behind breastbone
• worse when you lie down at night
• worse when you bend over

Have you been hitting the booze or taking 'acidic' tablets, e.g. aspirin, ibuprofen?
— no / yes →

gastritis
• when blood vomited up, much more likely to look like coffee grounds than fresh blood

Have you an alcohol problem or liver trouble?
— no / yes →

oesophageal varices
• if burst, you are likely to vomit up a lot of fresh blood

Only rare causes left, e.g.

stomach cancer
• often vague symptoms, e.g. fullness, indigestion, for months before diagnosis suspected
• may suddenly go off certain foods
• weight loss

Regardless of the possible cause, if you vomit up more than a cupful of blood, vomit up blood more than once, or feel faint or ill as well, then go to hospital without delay. Note also: vomited blood can look like 'coffee grounds'.

Swallowed blood Blood from a nosebleed or, less commonly, blood coughed up from the lungs can be swallowed and then vomited back up again.

Treatment If it's obviously blood you've swallowed from a nosebleed, then you have nothing to worry about. If it's blood you've been coughing up, then you need to look at the 'Blood in spit' flow chart (p. 34).

Mallory–Weiss tear A violent retch during vomiting can tear a blood vessel in the stomach or gullet, causing leakage of blood. This is then brought up in the next vomit.

Treatment If it's a small amount of blood (say less than a cupful) mixed in with the vomit, and it happens only once, and you otherwise feel reasonably OK (apart from the vomiting, of course), then there's nothing to worry about. But if it's more than this, it keeps happening, or you feel very ill, then you could have lost a significant amount of blood. Your best bet is to go to casualty as soon as possible.

Gastritis Overdoing the alcohol (especially binge drinking), or using a lot of 'acidic' tablets like ibuprofen or aspirin, can inflame the stomach lining. This is called gastritis, and it can cause bleeding, just like it does in reflux oesophagitis (see below).

Treatment You'll need checking over at the hospital and will probably be given a course of acid-suppressant treatment – and, in the future, you'll need to avoid whatever brought it on in the first place.

Duodenal ulcer This is explained in the 'Acidity/duodenal ulcer' part of the 'Abdominal pain – recurrent' section (p. 10) and also the 'Duodenal or gastric ulcer' part of the 'Indigestion' section (p. 78). A duodenal ulcer can bleed, leading to blood being vomited – or the blood may appear in your motions as 'melaena' (black, tarry, very smelly motions, which are partially digested blood). The problem may be caused or aggravated by some 'insult' to your guts – such as an alcoholic binge or taking acidic tablets like ibuprofen.

Treatment These types of bleeds are usually bad enough to need hospital treatment. You may well end up on acid-suppressant drugs for life. For other measures you can take to prevent trouble in the future, see the 'Abdominal pain – recurrent' (p. 10) and 'Indigestion' (p. 78) sections.

Reflux oesophagitis This is explained in the 'Indigestion' section (p. 78). If the lining of the gullet gets very inflamed, it may leak blood, which can be vomited up. It can pass out the other end too, as 'melaena' (see above).

Treatment You're likely to need hospital tests and treatment, so go to casualty. Once sorted out, you can then look at a number of areas you can tweak to try to prevent trouble in the future – these are explained in the 'Indigestion' section (p. 78). If you've had a serious bleed caused by reflux oesophagitis, then you may be put on an acid-suppressant drug indefinitely.

Oesophageal varices These are huge varicose veins – bloated blood vessels – in your gullet. When one pops, it causes dramatic bleeding.

Treatment There won't be much doubt about what to do in this situation: get an ambulance.

Other rare problems There are a few medical rarities which might cause this symptom, such as stomach cancer. The cancer can eat its way into a blood vessel; the leaked blood is then vomited up. Thankfully, this is very, very unlikely under the age of 50.

Treatment Most rare problems are likely to cause a lot of blood in the vomit, so hospital treatment is needed urgently. If the blood is only a small amount and only happens from time to time, consult your doctor.

Vulval and groin lumps and swellings

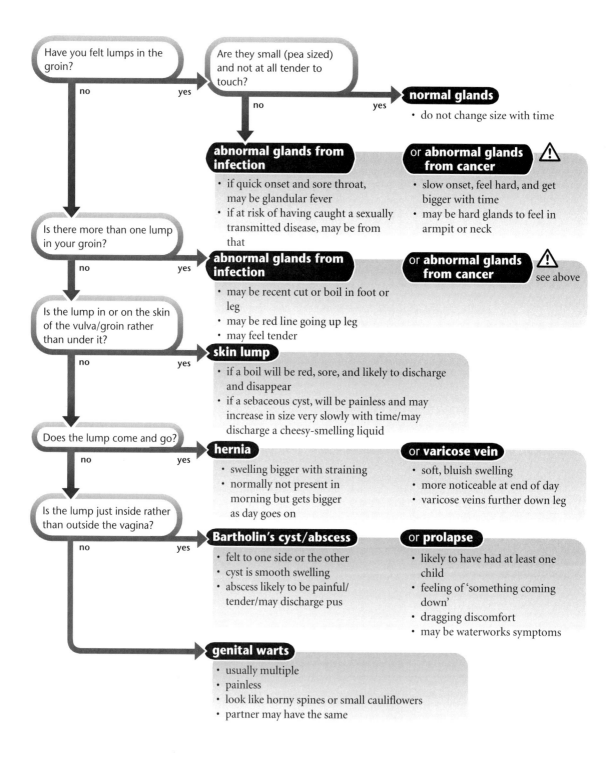

Have you felt lumps in the groin? — **no** / **yes**

Are they small (pea sized) and not at all tender to touch? — **no** / **yes**

normal glands
- do not change size with time

abnormal glands from infection
- if quick onset and sore throat, may be glandular fever
- if at risk of having caught a sexually transmitted disease, may be from that

or abnormal glands from cancer ⚠
- slow onset, feel hard, and get bigger with time
- may be hard glands to feel in armpit or neck

Is there more than one lump in your groin? — **no** / **yes**

abnormal glands from infection
- may be recent cut or boil in foot or leg
- may be red line going up leg
- may feel tender

or abnormal glands from cancer ⚠
see above

Is the lump in or on the skin of the vulva/groin rather than under it? — **no** / **yes**

skin lump
- if a boil will be red, sore, and likely to discharge and disappear
- if a sebaceous cyst, will be painless and may increase in size very slowly with time/may discharge a cheesy-smelling liquid

Does the lump come and go? — **no** / **yes**

hernia
- swelling bigger with straining
- normally not present in morning but gets bigger as day goes on

or varicose vein
- soft, bluish swelling
- more noticeable at end of day
- varicose veins further down leg

Is the lump just inside rather than outside the vagina? — **no** / **yes**

Bartholin's cyst/abscess
- felt to one side or the other
- cyst is smooth swelling
- abscess likely to be painful/tender/may discharge pus

or prolapse
- likely to have had at least one child
- feeling of 'something coming down'
- dragging discomfort
- may be waterworks symptoms

genital warts
- usually multiple
- painless
- look like horny spines or small cauliflowers
- partner may have the same

Normal glands Glands are found in various parts of the body – particularly the neck, the armpits, and the groin. They are a part of your immune system, which helps fight off infections. If you're slim, it's quite normal to be able to feel these glands as pea-sized, non-tender lumps which stay roughly the same size most of the time.

Treatment Being able to feel these glands is entirely normal, so no treatment is needed.

Abnormal glands from infection Sometimes, the 'normal' glands in the groin (described above) can swell because a germ has got into your body. Causes include bugs which enter the body near the groin (such as an infected cut on the leg or a sexually transmitted disease) or other infections which make all the glands swell (like glandular fever – see the 'General infection' part of the 'Swollen glands' section, p. 142).

Treatment This obviously needs careful checking by your GP, who will treat the infection which has made the glands swell.

Skin lump (various types) The skin can develop a variety of different lumps, and any of these can be found in the groin. Especially common are sebaceous cysts (blocked glands which produce the grease on our skin), lipomas (small collections of fat), and boils or abscesses (infections causing a small swelling full of pus).

Treatment Most of these swellings are totally harmless and are best left alone. If they're caused by infection, they normally enlarge and become tender, in which case you may need either antibiotics or the swelling lancing – speak to your GP. Recurrent boils in your groin area are occasionally caused by diabetes. If you want this possibility checked out, take a urine specimen to your GP or practice nurse for testing.

Genital warts These are explained, and their treatment outlined, in the 'Vulval irritation and/or sores' section (p. 158).

Varicose vein A varicose vein is a swollen, twisting vein, usually found in the leg. Severe varicose veins can start from the groin, producing a noticeable swelling – the rest of the vein may be more difficult to feel.

Treatment Varicose veins rarely cause any problems. If they ache or look terrible, they can be treated either with a tight stocking or with an operation – but they often tend to come back again after surgery, especially if you're planning future pregnancies, which tend to aggravate the problem. If you can't just put up with them, discuss the problem with your GP.

Bartholin's cyst/abscess A gland (Bartholin's gland) which produces small amounts of natural lubricant in the front passage ('vulva') can sometimes get blocked. This results in a swelling, or 'cyst'. If the cyst gets infected, it becomes painful and fills with pus (a Bartholin's abscess).

Treatment A small cyst which doesn't bother you is safe to leave alone. Larger or troublesome cysts need a small operation, so see your GP, who will probably refer you to a gynaecologist – though it's worth bearing in mind that the cyst may come back, even after surgery. A Bartholin's abscess will require either antibiotics (if in its early stages) or an operation (if it's full of pus) – so see your GP asap.

Prolapse A prolapse means that an internal organ is hanging down below it's normal position, usually because of muscular weakness – in turn, usually the result of previous childbirth. Prolapse may affect the bladder, the womb, or the back passage. You're more likely to have the sensation of a lump 'down below' than actually feel or see one – though some severe prolapses can be seen as a lump at the vulva.

Treatment Self-help measures may sort out a mild prolapse. Stopping smoking and sorting out constipation (to avoid coughing or straining aggravating the prolapse), and losing weight (being overweight puts a strain on the pelvic muscles), may relieve the problem. Pelvic floor exercises – such as deliberately stopping your flow of urine on and off when you pass water – may help, although you may have to wait many weeks before you notice much difference. If these measures don't help, or the problem is severe or seems to be upsetting your waterworks, then see your GP – she'll discuss the options for further treatment, which may include physiotherapy or seeing a gynaecologist for possible surgery (but she may well suggest delaying surgery until you're sure you've completed your family).

Hernia This is a bulge of the bowel through a muscle weakness.

Treatment The only effective treatment for a hernia is an operation, so see your GP to confirm this is the problem and to book an appointment with a surgeon. Rarely, a hernia can strangulate. This means that it gets throttled by the surrounding muscles, resulting in the swelling becoming very tender, hard, and 'irreducible' – it doesn't disappear with firm pressure or on lying down. A strangulated hernia will also block the bowel, causing pain, swelling of the abdomen, and vomiting. If you think your hernia is strangulating then get to the hospital asap.

Abnormal glands from cancer Very rarely, serious diseases (such as lymph gland cancers) can make the glands in the groin slowly get larger, and may affect other glands as well.

Treatment See your GP. If she suspects a serious cause like cancer, she'll refer you urgently to a hospital specialist.

Vulval irritation and/or sores

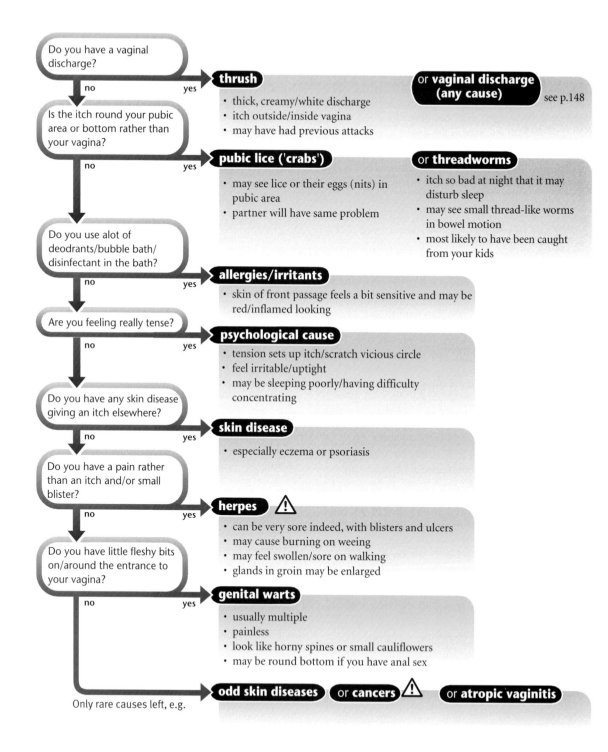

Do you have a vaginal discharge?

no | **yes**

thrush
- thick, creamy/white discharge
- itch outside/inside vagina
- may have had previous attacks

or **vaginal discharge (any cause)** see p.148

Is the itch round your pubic area or bottom rather than your vagina?

no | **yes**

pubic lice ('crabs')
- may see lice or their eggs (nits) in pubic area
- partner will have same problem

or **threadworms**
- itch so bad at night that it may disturb sleep
- may see small thread-like worms in bowel motion
- most likely to have been caught from your kids

Do you use alot of deodrants/bubble bath/disinfectant in the bath?

no | **yes**

allergies/irritants
- skin of front passage feels a bit sensitive and may be red/inflamed looking

Are you feeling really tense?

no | **yes**

psychological cause
- tension sets up itch/scratch vicious circle
- feel irritable/uptight
- may be sleeping poorly/having difficulty concentrating

Do you have any skin disease giving an itch elsewhere?

no | **yes**

skin disease
- especially eczema or psoriasis

Do you have a pain rather than an itch and/or small blister?

no | **yes**

herpes ⚠️
- can be very sore indeed, with blisters and ulcers
- may cause burning on weeing
- may feel swollen/sore on walking
- glands in groin may be enlarged

Do you have little fleshy bits on/around the entrance to your vagina?

no | **yes**

genital warts
- usually multiple
- painless
- look like horny spines or small cauliflowers
- may be round bottom if you have anal sex

Only rare causes left, e.g.

odd skin diseases or **cancers** ⚠️ or **atropic vaginitis**

Thrush This is caused by a fungus called 'Candida', which lives in the vaginas of many women without causing any symptoms at all. If it multiplies and spreads then it causes the familiar itching and discharge – this may happen after a course of antibiotics, during pregnancy, or for no particular reason at all. Some women get repeated attacks.

Treatment The jury's still out as to whether natual yoghurt is really effective – it probably just helps by cooling the area. Thrush is easily treated with pessaries, cream, or a tablet, all of which can be bought over the counter. If you get frequent attacks, don't overdo the washing and avoid vaginal deodorants, bubble baths, scented soaps, antiseptics, tights, synthetic underwear, and tight clothing as these tend to aggravate the problem. It's worth seeing your GP if all else fails – she'll confirm that the problem really is thrush (be prepared for an examination, though if it seems very likely to be thrush then most doctors will give you the treatment for this and only examine you if it doesn't work) and she may give you larger supplies of treatment to use when necessary, or as a preventive measure if your attacks tend to come with your periods. It's only worth your partner getting treatment if he has an itchy penis, in which case he can use some of your cream – thrush isn't usually passed on through sex.

Allergies/irritants The skin around the front passage (vulva) is very sensitive. It can be irritated by, or become allergic to, chemicals (like bath additives) or materials (such as the lubricants or rubber of condoms). These reactions cause itching.

Treatment In the short term, an anti-inflammatory cream like hydrocortisone 1% (available from the chemist) will ease the problem. The cure lies in working out whatever is triggering the reaction and avoiding it in future. If you think it might be condoms, try a low-allergy ('hypoallergenic') sort.

Vaginal discharge Any discharge from the vagina can irritate the vulva – for more details, see the 'Vaginal discharge' section (p. 148).

Herpes This is an infection caused by a virus, which results in blisters and ulcers on the genitals. There are two sorts: one which affects the genitals (passed on by having sex with an infected partner) and another which causes cold sores. Both can cause sores in the vagina or on the vulva (for example, cold sores can infect the genitals via oral sex). The body does not totally get rid of the herpes virus, even if you've been given treatment. Because of this, it can come back – you've about a 50/50 chance of future attacks, although these won't be as bad as the first one and they tend to get less frequent as time goes on.

Treatment Go to a department of genito-urinary medicine ('special clinic') asap, and take your partner too. Most hospitals have these clinics which specialize in sexually transmitted diseases – usually you just have to phone up to arrange an appointment. You'll receive treatment – usually tablets in this case – and be checked for any other sexually transmitted infections. If there's going to be a delay before you can be seen, speak to your GP – she may be able to start you off on treatment while you're waiting for your appointment. If you get attacks in the future, your GP or the doctors at the clinic will give you a cream to use. Very frequent attacks can sometimes be helped by taking tablets regularly for a while. It's worth getting your partner to wear condoms once you know you've had herpes, otherwise you risk spreading the infection to him. You need to do this even if you're not having an attack because the virus can be there without you realizing it. It's a good idea to avoid nude sunbathing, as this can bring on an attack. If you're pregnant and unlucky enough to get herpes when you're due, you'll need a Caesarean section, otherwise your baby might get infected during the delivery.

Pubic lice/threadworms Pubic lice (tiny creepy crawlies, also known as 'crabs') and threadworms (small thread-like worms, which usually live around the back passage) can both cause itching 'down below'.

Treatment See your GP to confirm the problem and get treatment. Pubic lice are passed on through sex, so it's probably worth getting checked for other infections.

Skin disease Any itchy skin disease – such as eczema – may cause irritation of your vulva. For more information, see the 'Eczema' part of the 'Itchy skin' section (p. 84).

Genital warts These are caused by viruses and are usually passed on through sex.

Treatment Go to the local 'special clinic' (see above), where you'll get treatment and be checked out for other sexually transmitted diseases. Take your partner too and make sure he wears a condom until your warts have been cured.

Psychological Tension can cause itching, making you scratch, leading to inflamed skin and more itching. Sexual frustration or a dislike of sex can cause similar symptoms.

Treatment For the treatment of tension, see the 'Feeling tense' section (p. 64). Otherwise, your GP or a psychosexual therapist (a 'sexpert') may be able to help.

Rare causes Atrophic vaginitis (the thinning of the skin of the vagina after the menopause), diabetes, unusual or tropical diseases, odd skin diseases, and cancers or precancerous changes can, very rarely, cause ulcers or irritation.

Treatment You're very unlikely to have any of these – if you're worried, see your GP.

Waterworks problems

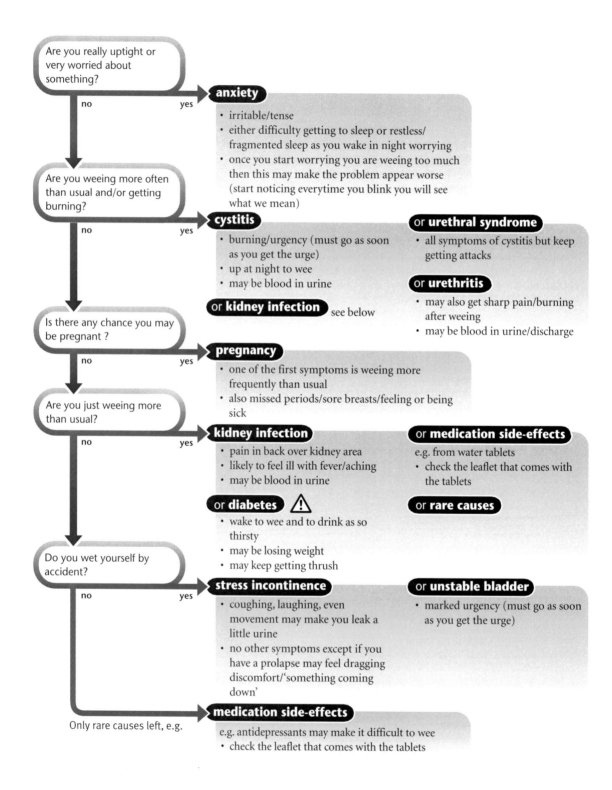

Are you really uptight or very worried about something?

no → yes →

anxiety
- irritable/tense
- either difficulty getting to sleep or restless/fragmented sleep as you wake in night worrying
- once you start worrying you are weeing too much then this may make the problem appear worse (start noticing everytime you blink you will see what we mean)

Are you weeing more often than usual and/or getting burning?

no → yes →

cystitis
- burning/urgency (must go as soon as you get the urge)
- up at night to wee
- may be blood in urine

or kidney infection see below

or urethral syndrome
- all symptoms of cystitis but keep getting attacks

or urethritis
- may also get sharp pain/burning after weeing
- may be blood in urine/discharge

Is there any chance you may be pregnant ?

no → yes →

pregnancy
- one of the first symptoms is weeing more frequently than usual
- also missed periods/sore breasts/feeling or being sick

Are you just weeing more than usual?

no → yes →

kidney infection
- pain in back over kidney area
- likely to feel ill with fever/aching
- may be blood in urine

or medication side-effects
e.g. from water tablets
- check the leaflet that comes with the tablets

or diabetes ⚠
- wake to wee and to drink as so thirsty
- may be losing weight
- may keep getting thrush

or rare causes

Do you wet yourself by accident?

no → yes →

stress incontinence
- coughing, laughing, even movement may make you leak a little urine
- no other symptoms except if you have a prolapse may feel dragging discomfort/'something coming down'

or unstable bladder
- marked urgency (must go as soon as you get the urge)

Only rare causes left, e.g.

medication side-effects
e.g. antidepressants may make it difficult to wee
- check the leaflet that comes with the tablets

Cystitis Infections of the bladder are common in women because the tube which you pass water through (the urethra) is very short, so germs can easily get in, causing 'cystitis'. These infections aren't actually sexually transmitted, but intercourse can bring on an attack. Some women get repeated episodes of cystitis.

Treatment You may be able to cure cystitis yourself by drinking plenty of fluids or trying an over-the-counter remedy. Otherwise, contact your GP – she may prescribe you antibiotics. If you get repeated attacks, try some simple self-help remedies like a high fluid intake and making sure you empty your bladder before and after intercourse. But if you're getting nowhere, see your GP – you may need further tests to see if there is an underlying cause (which is very unusual), or she may prescribe you antibiotics to prevent the problem or to nip it in the bud when it happens.

Anxiety The bladder is a muscular bag which collects your urine until you're ready to pass it. If you're uptight, the bladder tenses up, so it can't hold as much urine as usual. Being stressed also makes the bladder muscle twitchy, which will make you want to keep running to the loo. You'll have noticed this when you've felt nervous about something – the same thing can happen if you're very cold.

Treatment This is a normal reaction so no treatment is needed. You might get persistent trouble if you're feeling anxious all the time – try the techniques explained in the 'Anxiety' part of the 'Feeling tense' (p. 64) and 'Palpitations' (p. 116) sections.

Urethral syndrome This produces the symptoms of cystitis but without there being any obvious germ to explain it. Doctors don't agree on the cause – some view it as a sign of stress or depression and others believe it's caused by a 'hidden' infection.

Treatment As the cause is unknown, it's difficult to treat. Discuss the situation with your GP (and take a urine specimen) so she can check there's no other reason for the symptoms. Dietary changes and a high fluid intake sometimes help; if you think stress or depression might be the cause, check the 'Feeling down' (p. 62) and 'Feeling tense' (p. 64) sections.

Pregnancy Passing urine more frequently is an early sign of pregnancy – it's quite normal and so needs no treatment.

Stress incontinence This is a leakage of urine on coughing, moving, laughing, and so on. It's caused by a weakness of the muscles which support the bladder – and so tends to be more common in women who've had children, as childbirth tends to stretch or damage these muscles. Sometimes the muscle weakness results in a 'prolapse', in which one of the pelvic organs (such as the womb or bladder) drops down from its normal position.

Treatment First, sort out any aggravating factors such as overweight (which puts pressure on the bladder) and smoking (coughing stretches the muscles supporting the bladder). The next step is pelvic floor exercises to tone up the muscles – you can learn these from books or from your GP or practice nurse. They can take some months to work, but see your GP if you're getting nowhere – you may need to see a gynaecologist with a view to surgery, especially if you have a bad prolapse.

Unstable bladder This means the bladder empties when you're not expecting it to so you have to rush to the loo – and you might even wet yourself.

Treatment Your GP will need to confirm this is the likely cause of your symptoms, so make an appointment and take a urine specimen. Treatment involves bladder retraining (teaching your bladder to 'accept' increasingly larger volumes of urine). Medication may help too.

Urethritis This is an infection of the urethra (see above) which is passed on through sex. Examples of this type of infection are chlamydia and gonorrhoea.

Treatment Go to a department of genito-urinary medicine ('special clinic'). Most hospitals have these clinics which specialize in sexually transmitted diseases – usually you just have to phone up to arrange an appointment. There you will be checked out for other sexually transmitted diseases and given any necessary treatment – try to get your partner to go too as he'll also need checking over.

Kidney infection This is caused by a germ getting into your kidney (usually via the bladder). Further details are given in the 'Back pain' section (p. 24).

Medication side-effect Some prescribed treatments, such as antidepressants, can occasionally make it difficult to wee properly; others (commonly known as 'water tablets') make you wee more, though you're unlikely to be on these.

Treatment If you think your medication is upsetting your waterworks, see your GP.

Diabetes This is explained, and its treatment outlined, in the 'Weight-loss' section (p. 164)

Other rare causes A few small-print problems, such as stones in your bladder, a narrowing of your urethra (water passage), and swellings on your ovaries or womb pressing on your bladder, can also affect your waterworks.

Treatment It's unlikely that any of these are the cause of your problems, but if you're concerned, see your GP.

Weight gain

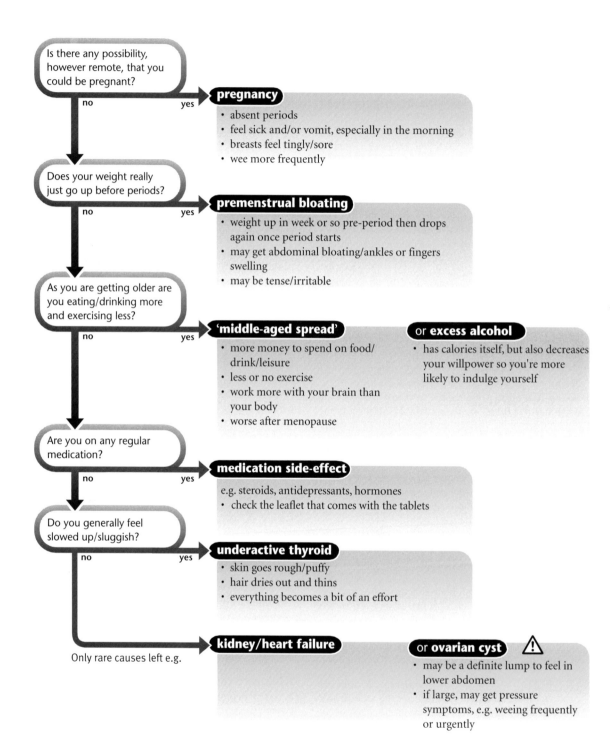

Is there any possibility, however remote, that you could be pregnant?

no / yes

pregnancy
- absent periods
- feel sick and/or vomit, especially in the morning
- breasts feel tingly/sore
- wee more frequently

Does your weight really just go up before periods?

no / yes

premenstrual bloating
- weight up in week or so pre-period then drops again once period starts
- may get abdominal bloating/ankles or fingers swelling
- may be tense/irritable

As you are getting older are you eating/drinking more and exercising less?

no / yes

'middle-aged spread'
- more money to spend on food/drink/leisure
- less or no exercise
- work more with your brain than your body
- worse after menopause

or excess alcohol
- has calories itself, but also decreases your willpower so you're more likely to indulge yourself

Are you on any regular medication?

no / yes

medication side-effect
e.g. steroids, antidepressants, hormones
- check the leaflet that comes with the tablets

Do you generally feel slowed up/sluggish?

no / yes

underactive thyroid
- skin goes rough/puffy
- hair dries out and thins
- everything becomes a bit of an effort

Only rare causes left e.g.

kidney/heart failure

or ovarian cyst
- may be a definite lump to feel in lower abdomen
- if large, may get pressure symptoms, e.g. weeing frequently or urgently

'Middle-aged spread' Far and away the commonest cause of weight gain is a lousy lifestyle which leads to you piling on the pounds. There's nothing complicated about working out how and why the weight goes on. If you take in more fuel (food and drink) than you burn off (in exercise) then the surplus is stored – in the form of fat. As you get older, your metabolism – the rate at which you use up the fuel – slows down. The hormone changes of the menopause can also affect your metabolism, which may aggravate the problem. So, to keep the same weight, you need to eat less or exercise more. Usually, the opposite happens, so the dreaded middle-aged spread develops.

Treatment There's no easy answer, although thousands are advertised – most miracle cures are simply there to make a fast buck. The only effective way to sort out your weight in the long term is to alter your lifestyle – this means eating more healthily and taking more exercise. You don't need to go on a crash diet. Healthy eating is the rule with plenty of fruit, fresh vegetables, fibre, white meat, and fish rather than fast and junk foods, red meat, cakes, and so on – advice you're likely to have heard before. Sensible diet sheets are readily available at the chemist's and your doctor's. Aim for a steady weight loss and consider joining a group if you're very fat or having real problems shedding the excessive pounds. Exercise regularly and gradually build up the amount you do – use your common sense and don't go hell for leather from day one, as sudden and extreme exercise can be bad for the unfit body. There's very little point seeing your GP for a magic bullet, as drug treatment is not usually viewed as a sensible or effective way to slim down. She may be able to point you in the direction of a good diet or slimming group, and can advise you about exercise, though. And if you're only a few pounds overweight, don't get too obsessed about it as it probably isn't that bad for you – and you still need to enjoy life.

Pregnancy You won't be surprised to hear that you tend to put on weight during pregnancy and that this is, of course, perfectly normal.

Premenstrual It's quite normal to feel bloated and retain a little fluid before a period – for further details, see the 'Abdominal swelling or bloating' section (p. 12).

Excess alcohol Alcohol is full of calories – so if you've read the information about 'middle-aged spread', above, you'll be able to work out why drinking too much will pile on the weight. If you're developing a serious alcohol problem, you can end up seriously ill and retaining a lot of fluid, which will also make you gain weight.

Treatment Cut down your intake. And if you think you have a major problem, see your GP as you will need a careful check-up, advice on how to stop drinking, and maybe the help of a specialist.

Medication side-effect Some treatments, such as antidepressants, migraine-preventers, some hormone treatments, and steroids, can cause weight gain as a side-effect. But the Pill – contrary to popular belief – does not cause this problem.

Treatment Check the leaflet that comes with your medication to see if weight gain is a side-effect. If so, discuss the situation with your GP.

Underactive thyroid The thyroid gland sits in the front of your neck and produces a hormone, 'thyroxine', which controls your metabolism. If it becomes underactive, it stops producing enough thyroxine, so your metabolism slows up. Weight gain is one effect of this.

Treatment See your GP. She will take a blood test if she thinks you may have an underactive thyroid. It's easily treated with tablets, which you'll have to take for the rest of your life.

Other medical illness There are a few rarities which can cause weight gain, such as a large ovarian cyst, hormone problems, and heart and kidney failure.

Treatment The chances that any of these problems will reveal themselves by making you put on weight are virtually zero (an ovarian cyst usually produces other symptoms such as pain or swelling). If your GP thinks it's necessary, she'll run some tests.

Weight loss

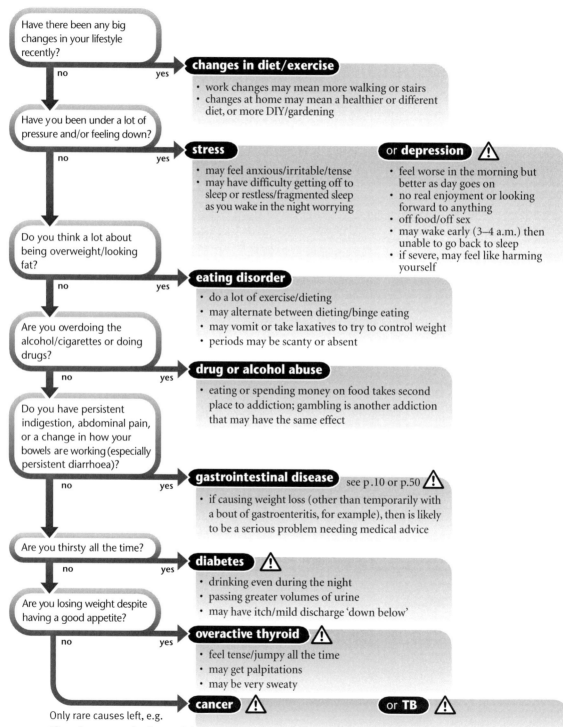

Have there been any big changes in your lifestyle recently?

no → yes →

changes in diet/exercise
- work changes may mean more walking or stairs
- changes at home may mean a healthier or different diet, or more DIY/gardening

Have you been under a lot of pressure and/or feeling down?

no → yes →

stress
- may feel anxious/irritable/tense
- may have difficulty getting off to sleep or restless/fragmented sleep as you wake in the night worrying

or depression ⚠
- feel worse in the morning but better as day goes on
- no real enjoyment or looking forward to anything
- off food/off sex
- may wake early (3–4 a.m.) then unable to go back to sleep
- if severe, may feel like harming yourself

Do you think a lot about being overweight/looking fat?

no → yes →

eating disorder
- do a lot of exercise/dieting
- may alternate between dieting/binge eating
- may vomit or take laxatives to try to control weight
- periods may be scanty or absent

Are you overdoing the alcohol/cigarettes or doing drugs?

no → yes →

drug or alcohol abuse
- eating or spending money on food takes second place to addiction; gambling is another addiction that may have the same effect

Do you have persistent indigestion, abdominal pain, or a change in how your bowels are working (especially persistent diarrhoea)?

no → yes →

gastrointestinal disease see p.10 or p.50 ⚠
- if causing weight loss (other than temporarily with a bout of gastroenteritis, for example), then is likely to be a serious problem needing medical advice

Are you thirsty all the time?

no → yes →

diabetes ⚠
- drinking even during the night
- passing greater volumes of urine
- may have itch/mild discharge 'down below'

Are you losing weight despite having a good appetite?

no → yes →

overactive thyroid ⚠
- feel tense/jumpy all the time
- may get palpitations
- may be very sweaty

cancer ⚠   **or TB** ⚠

Only rare causes left, e.g.

⚠ If you have started to lose weight and feel very thirsty, you may be developing diabetes, and need to seek medical advice quickly.

Changes in diet/exercise There is normally a balance between the fuel you put into your body (in other words, what you eat) and the fuel you burn off (how much exercise you do). If this balance is shifted, the result will be a change in weight – so you'll tend to slim down if you exercise more or eat less.

Treatment Changes in weight of this sort are obviously normal – and good for your health if you were overweight to begin with.

Stress Being uptight all the time is another way of burning up energy; tension also tends to take away the appetite. The result: weight loss.

Treatment This is covered elsewhere – particularly in the 'Anxiety state' part of the 'Feeling tense' section (p. 64) and the 'Anxiety' part of the 'Palpitations' section (p. 116).

Depression Feeling very down often affects the appetite. Feeling tense may be a part of depression, too, and this will aggravate your weight loss. Depression is explained in more detail, and its treatment outlined, in the 'Feeling down' section (p. 62).

Eating disorder This term covers illnesses like anorexia nervosa (in which the sufferer is underweight and has a profound fear of getting fat) and bulimia nervosa (in which there is also a preoccupation with weight, together with food binges). There is a lot of overlap between the two and vomiting can be a feature of both (usually via a finger down the throat). It's difficult to know what causes these problems – it's probably a combination of cultural pressures (such as the view that 'thinness' is attractive), personality traits, your job (it's more common, for example, in models and athletes), and heredity (these illnesses sometimes run in families).

Treatment If you suffer from bulimia, it's important to focus on overcoming the eating problem rather than losing weight. So avoid strict dieting and try to eat regularly – this helps stop the cycle of bingeing. You may find it helps to keep a diary of the food you eat together with notes about your feelings at the time, as this will enable you to spot problem areas. There are a number of self-help books available which can be very useful. If you're getting nowhere, see your GP for further treatment – you should certainly do this if you're suffering from anorexia, as this illness can become very severe indeed. Some women are reluctant to seek help, perhaps because they don't accept that they have an illness, feel guilty about it, or think that nothing can be done. It's important to overcome these feelings – and if friends or relatives are telling you that you have a problem, it's worth letting them persuade you to see a doctor.

Drug or alcohol abuse Overdoing the alcohol or illicit substances can make you shed weight in a number of ways. It leads to a chaotic lifestyle, with eating properly being low on your list of priorities; it can cause anxiety and depression; it can mess up your finances so you can't afford proper meals; it can cause illnesses (like hepatitis); and some drugs (such as amphetamines) simply burn off the calories.

Treatment Cut down – or better still, stop – the substance abuse and get a grip on your lifestyle. If you find it difficult and want help, check out your local drug or alcohol services (try the Citizen's Advice Bureau or the phone directory) or see your GP.

Gastrointestinal disease Your gastrointestinal tract starts at your mouth and ends at your back passage. Problems anywhere in between can make you lose weight. Examples include duodenal ulcer (which stops you eating properly – see the 'Acidity/duodenal ulcer' part of the 'Abdominal pain – recurrent' section, p. 10) and inflammatory bowel disease or malabsorption (in which your food passes out as diarrhoea and so doesn't get absorbed into your system – see the 'Diarrhoea' section, p. 50).

Treatment If you have a gut problem severe enough to make you lose weight, you need to see your GP.

Diabetes If your body fails to produce enough of the chemical 'insulin', your blood sugar starts ro rise – this is diabetes. It's quite common, affecting one in 100 people, but no one knows exactly why it happens. When it first develops – before you realize you're suffering from it – it can cause a number of symptoms, including weight loss.

Treatment See your GP asap – and take a specimen of wee with you, as she'll want to test this. If it does turn out that you have diabetes, you'll need a special diet, probably with either tablets or insulin injections.

Overactive thyroid Weight loss is one of the many symptoms an overactive thyroid causes. For further details and advice about treatment, see the 'Excess sweating' section (p. 58).

Medical rarities Some small-print medical conditions, such as cancer, TB, and AIDS, can cause dramatic weight loss, although there are usually lots of other symptoms which make it quite obvious that you're seriously ill.

Treatment If you think you might have one of these problems, see your GP asap.

Part Three

Having it all

When it comes to healthy living, it might seem that women have it all already, including a six-year advantage over blokes in average lifespan (80 as opposed to 74 years). That said, however, no woman worth her salt doesn't spend a lot of time and money trying to improve on nature.

Whatever it is you want to do – diet, exercise, get fit, stay slim, have the perfect sex life/career/skin/bust/bottom/thighs – and the list is endless, someone out there will be happy to give you advice and sell you something to help. There is just so much information it is hard to get at the truth in amongst all the hype.

The media long ago realized that, as far as women are concerned, health sells. But with so many people keen to get in on the act, there's enormous pressure to package old news in new ways, just to get it off the bookshelves and into your home. This is particularly true of diets – with 60% of young women in one survey admitting to dieting in the past year, even though only 9% were clinically overweight, it's a marketer's dream.

Doctors add to the confusion, with conflicting opinions and advice and sudden complete changes in medical opinion that happen often enough to make you wonder if anyone really knows what they're talking about. For example, how would you feel if for years you had been eating loads of fruit and veg – and spending a fortune on toilet paper – thinking you were helping to prevent cancer of the bowel, only to be suddenly told that doctors no longer believed a high fibre diet had any effect on this? Gutted. Yet that happened recently and it would be no surprise if the view changed back again in the future.

So giving advice can be tricky, but that is not going to stop us giving you some! Please note where we are coming from:

- We are not experts but we all deal with women's health every day of the week – and spend a lot of time looking at medical advances. Naturally, not everyone is going to agree with our suggestions, but they are based on a good consensus of 'best medical practice'.

- We're trained to interpret medical research, so we have a much better chance than most of spotting an iffy bit of hype.

- We don't mind if you follow our advice or not (although we'd really like you to be around long enough to buy future editions of this book).

- We're aware that you have more than enough to worry about without bothering about improving areas of your health that would involve an awful lot of hassle for very little benefit.

- Risk factors are just that – factors which increase your risk/chances of getting a disease in the future. However, there are no certainties. You can have all the risks and not get the disease or you can have no risks at all and still get it. Life just isn't fair sometimes.

- Most of the risk factors we're going to be talking about – cigarettes, stress, too much drink, and so on – can harm you in the short term too. The effects may be more subtle – dull, lank hair, blotchy skin, feeling constantly knackered – but they're still very real.

- Contrary to popular belief, doctors are not a frustrated bunch of killjoys. Life is for living and if something is fine in moderation, or even in excess, we'll say so. Life is as much about quality as quantity.

Which brings us neatly to the next bit – your guide to healthy living.

1. Do all (or nearly all) things in moderation.

Apart from smoking and doing drugs, there aren't many things that'll do you harm in moderation – and that includes chocolate! Even stress can be quite positive sometimes – there's nothing like a deadline to concentrate the mind. But, by the same token, there are some good things you can get too much of. Dieting is a case in point – no one starts off dieting with the aim of becoming anorexic, but with 10 times as many girls affected as blokes, and most of them in the younger age groups, it has to happen to someone. Even if you recover your weight and your mental health, it can leave you with osteoporosis (thinning of the bones) and other problems in later life.

Likewise, doctors have known for years that crash diets are bad for your body (apart from the fact that this doesn't teach you to eat healthily when you stop dieting). As if that wasn't enough, it now seems crash diets can adversely affect your brainpower too. Even exercise isn't immune – there's no one who shouldn't do any, but too much can stop your periods, damage your joints, and play havoc with your mental health. The same goes for looking after your health. Ignoring your health completely is the perfect way to kill yourself slowly, but hypochondriacs are likely to die younger than average. And while there are some kinds of health screening which are worthwhile (see below), you can do yourself psychological damage by dwelling too much on the results – even if they're normal.

2. Get fitter and slimmer – but don't be a stick insect.

There are lots of dangers associated with being very overweight – you're more likely to get heart disease, diabetes, and high blood pressure, as well as arthritis and other problems. There's also much more pressure on you as girls to keep your weight down – not least the inability of clothes designers to come up with anything over size 14 that doesn't look like a Day-Glo barrage balloon. Having said that, the media – especially the fashion world – would have you believe that anything over a size 6 just isn't sexy. Yet what's sexy about anorexia, when you feel constantly tired, guilty about eating a twiglet (even though you look like one), and spend so much of your time working out when you can next throw up that your can't hold down a relationship?

One-third of the working women in this country are overweight – yet average calories intakes are lower than ever. This is largely down to lack of exercise rather than some great conspiracy – we're rapidly turning into a nation of couch potatoes, who won't even walk to the corner shop when there's a pizza parlour just around the corner that will deliver. The logic is quite simple. Taking in more calories than you burn up means you'll put on weight, and using up more calories than you eat will mean you'll lose it.

Exercise is great for burning calories as well as for making you feel fitter, trimmer, and more energetic – it'll also reduce your chances of heart disease and osteoporosis, stave off anxiety and depression, and possibly help you to preserve your brain cells, so you get to keep your marbles in old age. On its own, though, it's hard to do enough exercise to counteract Mars bars on demand – so you need to get into a regime that combines regular exercise with a sensible, feasible eating plan.

So how regular is regular? Vigorous exercising – hard enough to get a bit sweaty and breathless – for about 20 minutes three times a week is about right. Gentler exercise, like walking, is pretty much as good if you do a bit more – say seven hours a week. Ideally, you should make exercise part of your everyday routine – get into the habit of taking the stairs rather than the lift, or follow the celebrity who set herself a Millennium promise never to use the car for journeys of under a mile. If that's not feasible, try and find an exercise you can enjoy – you're much more likely to stick to it if you do.

3. Eat a healthy diet – including some chocolate.

These days, there's so much information around about which foods are good for you and which aren't that you'd think you could find out easily what makes up a healthy diet. Needless to say, the opposite is probably true – if you waded through all the hype about the life-giving properties of food X or the dangers of food Y, you'd probably be so confused you'd never dare eat again! Part of the confusion comes from the fact that food fashions and opinions seem to change constantly – partly as new research emerges, but more commonly because someone's trying to flog another diet book.

Actually, the rules for a healthy diet are pretty simple – eat more of the good stuff (especially fruit and vegetables) and less of the bad (like sugar, fat, and highly refined foods). Here are a few simple guidelines:

- Eat 5–9 measures daily of fruit and vegetables (fresh, frozen, or canned).
- Eat 2–3 measures daily of dairy products (preferably low fat).
- Eat 4–8 measures daily of bread, cereals, rice, or pasta.
- Try and replace red meat with poultry, fish, or quorn/pulses when you can. Fish – especially fatty fish like mackerel, sardines, or salmon – is good for your heart.
- You don't need sweets, sugary drinks, cakes, pastry, or fry-ups, so keep them for special treats.
- You need a bit of fat in your diet, not least because it helps you absorb vitamins A, E, and D.
- You're much more likely to stick to a healthy diet if you enjoy it – so experiment with adding seeds, nuts, cheeses, etc. to salads to make them more interesting. Nuts and seeds are packed with vitamins, and the fat in them may actually protect your heart.
- And remember, chocolate can contribute to a healthy diet as it's good for the heart. For example, a 50 g bar of dark chocolate contains the same amount of antioxidant (which helps prevent heart disease) as two glasses of red wine.

4. Enjoy social drinking but don't get legless too often.

Here's the good news – women need to drink less than men to get the 'rewarding' effects of alcohol; and as far as alcohol goes, two or three units a day, four or five days a week isn't going to do you any harm, can be a useful social lubricant, and may well give you some protection against heart disease. Here's the bad news – firstly, while the recommended weekly limit is 14 units (one unit = a small glass of wine/half a pint of normal strength beer or lager/a single pub measure of spirits), the idea is to spread it out and *not* to take the lot all at once on an empty stomach on your girlie night out. Secondly, the fact that your recommended maximum alcohol intake is much lower than a bloke's isn't just a male conspiracy. Apart from being smaller, you have more body fat and less body water than a bloke of the same size – and since alcohol is concentrated in body water, that means you get drunk quicker and you knacker your liver faster too.

The fact that more than half the girls drinking over the recommended limit are single and under 25 is not surprising. These days, you'll probably spend large parts of your working day trying to prove you can match any bloke in the office – and there's bound to be pressure to prove you can match them in the pub too. But any binge – by which we mean more than seven units at a sitting – increases your risk of accidents, suicide attempts, and damage to your heart. You're also more likely to have unprotected sex or to be attacked – you may be a modern woman, but a couple of bottles of wine would play havoc with anyone's better judgement!

Of course, drinking more occasionally isn't going to do you much harm, but the more often you drink to excess, the more damage you do. Basically, the risks go up the further above the 14 units you are, until by the time you're averaging 35 units or more a week, you're likely to be in serious trouble.

5. Have as many orgasms as you can – but don't get pregnant unless you really want to.

Although all that panting may lead you to believe otherwise, sex is not particularly good exercise – even if you don't stick to the missionary position! However, regular sex does seem to be good at counteracting stress, as long as you don't end up frustrated.

And there's the rub. While girls may get just as much of a buzz as blokes from flirting and all the bits leading up to sex, they do take longer to climax when it comes to penetration. It's also much easier for girls to fake orgasm and, let's be frank, sometimes that just seems like the easiest option.

But sex without orgasm is at best less than satisfying, and at worst hardly worth the effort. So when you get a new relationship, it's well worth doing a little bit of gentle coaxing and education before he gets down to business – he'll find it a lot easier to satisfy you next time if he knows what turns you on. It also stands to reason that a regular partner is far more likely to invest the time and effort it takes to satisfy you – just one of many reasons for finding one partner and sticking to him.

These days, as long as you're responsible about contraception, there's little reason to worry about unwanted pregnancy. But it is worth remembering that even if you feel safer from pregnancy being on the Pill, you also want protection from sexually transmitted diseases. There's no law that says you can't use condoms too. It may also be worth 'forgetting' to mention to your partner that you're on the Pill – while blokes are, on the whole, very responsible about practising safe sex to avoid getting you pregnant, there are still a few of them who are pretty gung-ho about sexually transmitted diseases, and can't see the point of condoms if they know you're on the Pill.

It's also worth remembering that there's no such thing as truly 'safe' sex – only 'safer' sex. Even condoms don't offer 100% protection against sexually transmitted diseases – so casual sex is never a great idea. And while most sexually transmitted diseases (except herpes and, obviously, HIV) don't cause long-term problems for blokes if they're properly treated, the same doesn't apply to women.

6. Make time for yourself – because no one else will.

There's a good chance that you're one of the growing band of independent, financially self-sufficient women. Although you may still have to work harder than a bloke to prove yourself, at least you've got the chance to do just that. If all this sounds too good to be true, that's because, for many of you, it is. Getting yourself treated as an equal in a blokes' world can involve all sorts of sacrifices, mostly of time, and the great irony is that the more money you earn, the less time you have, as a rule, to enjoy it.

But the one thing you mustn't sacrifice is time for you. On the whole, women are really good at communicating and making and keeping friends – and there's good evidence that this keeps your stress levels and your blood pressure down and your general level of well-being up. Likewise, many of the 'bonding' things that you do are good for stress – having a facial or a massage, going to an aerobics class together, or just sitting around gossiping. That means that if you sacrifice time with your girlfriends because of pressures of work, you're losing out on two counts. What's more, it's probably counter-productive because there's good evidence that you're likely to work less effectively if you're too stressed and exhausted, and also you're less likely to have sex and orgasms as your libido gets shot to pieces.

7. Don't smoke – it's not big and it's not clever.

If you smoke, you're probably bored to death of hearing this message – but there's no doubt that smoking is the greatest self-inflicted health risk of the lot. Women in their teens and 20s smoke most, possibly because they think it'll keep them slim, then can't quit because they think it'll make them fat. In fact, if you do give up smoking you'll put on an average of 7 lb – but you can always lose it once you've stopped comfort eating, and the money you'll save on fags will pay for an awful lot of sessions at the gym.

On average, smoking will knock six years off your life – and will probably make the last few years pretty miserable as well. But even in the short term, smoking can open your pores, making your skin look blotchy and less smooth. It can give you bad breath and stained teeth, not to mention a permanent stale smell and less staying power on the dance floor.

There's no way of 'cheating' about being a smoker – cutting down means you don't really consider yourself an ex-smoker, and the fags are much more likely to creep up. Smoking low tar brands doesn't help either – you just drag deeper to try and get the same amount of nicotine into your lungs, so you end up with a particularly nasty form of cancer deeper inside your lungs. You need to just stop – but make sure you've planned your strategy for quitting, so you can avoid temptations and work out if you need help from one of the many forms of nicotine replacement on the market these days. If you do find yourself tempted, harden your resolve with the thought that, in time, you're reducing your risks to nearly those of a non-smoker – and saving yourself a packet!

8. Don't do drugs.

No one has ever shown that drugs are in any way good for you. Despite that, government research has shown that 45% of under 30s have taken an illegal drug at some point (15% in a given month), and that 10% have tried LSD, cocaine, or Ecstasy – which means we'd be completely unrealistic if we assumed that none of you reading this book had partaken.

If, despite advice to the contrary, you're determined to indulge, we would strongly advise you at least to choose your drugs carefully. Cannabis, for instance, has been found by the World Health Organization to be less addictive than alcohol or tobacco, and the odd spliff is more likely to land you in court than in hospital. Harder drugs are far less predictable – cocaine and crack can give you a heart attack, LSD can make you completely paranoid, Ecstasy, if taken in pregnancy, causes a high rate of heart/limb abnormalities in the baby, and if you get on to heroin you have 50/50 chance of being dead in 10 years. As if that wasn't enough, given the unscrupulous nature of dealers, they'll often cut your drugs with the kind of rubbish you wouldn't dream of touching otherwise.

If you think you have a drug problem or you're just finding it a bit harder than you thought to say no, get some help. Your GP can advise you, or you can refer yourself to the local drugs and alcohol advisory service.

9. Don't get too hung up on screening.

While there are certain types of screening (like having regular cervical smears) that are probably worth doing, getting too hung up on checking your bits can do more harm than good.

It may seem like a contradiction in terms to say screening can be bad for you – after all, surely if there's something wrong it's good to know early, and if there's nothing wrong it's just as good to be reassured. Right? Wrong. Screening isn't always harmless – it can lull you into a false sense of security (so if you do get symptoms you ignore them), reinforce bad habits, stop you relying on your own common sense, or put you through completely unnecessary worry.

For example, while it is certainly worthwhile having smear tests, you are far more likely to get an abnormal result which has to be checked out but which turns out to be nothing worth worrying about than you ever are to be one of the few women found to have treatable or preventable cancer.

In similar vein, one of the main reasons we no longer advise women to check their breasts obsessively every month is that breast self-examination revealed many lumps which turned out to be nothing to worry about, but which had to be investigated. This meant weeks of unnecessary angst and misery for hundreds, all to make sure we didn't miss the very rare lump they would have noticed anyway. That's especially the case if you're under 35, when non-cancerous lumps are far more common than nasty ones. Instead we now suggest that you get to be 'breast aware', getting to know what your breasts feel like normally when you're washing or dressing, so you can tell if something has changed.

The same goes for other things you're unlikely to suffer from, such as high blood pressure, heart attacks, or most forms of cancer. Living healthily is one thing – stressing yourself out for nothing is quite another.

Whatever you do, don't get pregnant . . .

Him How do you like your eggs in the morning?
Her Unfertilized.

An old joke, but one which no modern woman should ever have to lose sleep over. There's a wide choice of effective contraception and a society that (mostly) recognizes women as independent equals who have every right to do without a man if they want.

So why doesn't it feel that way? Why do so many women get pregnant when they don't want to? Sometimes, of course, contraception does fail – but it's more likely to if you haven't found the type that works best for you. This list may help you decide, although you should always follow the more detailed information you get from your doc.

- **The combined oral contraceptive pill** (the 'Pill'). The Pill works by stopping you from ovulating – the rationale being that if you don't produce an egg, it can't get fertilized. You usually take it for three weeks out of four, which protects you for all four weeks. It's up to 99% effective, and usually gives you light, painless, regular periods. It can fail if you are more than 12 hours late with a dose, vomit, have severe diarrhoea, or are taking other medicines. It can also rarely cause raised blood pressure and clots on your leg or lung.

- **The progesterone-only pill** (the 'minipill'). You take this pill at the same time every day, without a week off. It's up to 99% effective if you use it properly, but if you're more than three hours late with a dose you won't be protected for seven days. It can give you irregular periods and small cysts on the ovary, which are generally harmless but can be painful. You may be able to take it even if you have a medical condition that stops you being able to take the Pill itself.

- **The condom.** The only method of contraception that offers a good level of protection against sexually transmitted diseases (STDs). Some blokes don't like them (they may find them messy or tell you they reduce their pleasure) – but though they might tell you they can't use them because they don't fit, that's usually wishful thinking on their part! Female condoms do exist, but are more bulky.

- **The diaphragm.** This is a rubber cap that you get fitted initially by your doctor, then put in like a tampon before sex, and leave in for at least six hours afterwards. It's up to 96% effective, and some girls like it because it's natural (i.e. no hormones). It can make you more prone to cystitis.

- **The intrauterine contraceptive device or IUCD** (the coil). Often made of plastic wrapped with copper, the IUCD can be fitted without an anaesthetic and works until you have it taken out, up to five years later. It can cause heavier, more painful periods and can bring on pelvic infection, especially just after it's fitted. It also increases your risk of ectopic pregnancy (pregnancy outside the womb). Although it tends to be harder and more painful to fit if you haven't had a baby, there are smaller versions on the market which might suit you. Another type of coil releases small amounts of a hormone called progesterone and lasts for up to five years. It actually makes your periods lighter and less painful, but its size means it's rarely suitable if you haven't had a baby, and it can cause irregular bleeding for some months after it's put in.

- **Injection contraceptives** (also called depot contraception). A progesterone injection that protects you for up to three months. It's very effective, but it can cause heavy bleeding in the short term and stop you getting pregnant for several months after you stop it. If it does cause side-effects, you can't reverse them so you have to wait for them to wear off.

- **'Natural' methods** – coitus interruptus, safe period, and so on. Only recommended if you don't mind getting pregnant or like playing Russian roulette! The only natural method we know that works is having a young child at home – one young child, particularly if you are working as well, will mean you are simply too knackered to create a second.

- **Sterilization.** Don't even think about this if there's the slightest chance you might EVER want more kids. Reversal involves major surgery and very often doesn't work. If you're sure you want no more, and he has no objections, send him for the snip (a vasectomy).

Of course, just because you feel 'safer' from a pregnancy point of view, using a method of contraception other than condoms doesn't mean that you can't use them too. Indeed, it may be worth 'forgetting' to mention you're on the Pill – this saves all that negotiating about whether you really need to use a condom at all. Sadly, as mentioned previously, some blokes are pretty gung-ho about STDs – which could be because, as the old joke goes, God gave them a brain and a penis but only enough blood to supply one at a time. It could also be that blokes often don't get symptoms from STDs (except AIDS of course) and certainly don't get the same complications as women.

Finally, if you get taken short and, for whatever reason, have unprotected sex or a possible failure of contraception, then don't forget emergency contraception which really can help lock the stable door just before the horse bolts. Pill or minipill hormones (in much higher one-off doses) taken up to 72 hours after sex are very likely to be effective. An alternative is to have a coil (IUCD) fitted temporarily, this is very effective up to 5 days after one-off mid-cycle sex. If you ever need emergency contraception then ask your doc ASAP.

. . . Unless you really want to

Now, if you've followed the advice opposite, you won't have to think about having a baby until you've found Mr Perfect and the idea makes you go all weak and fluffy inside. Unlikely as that may seem to you now, chances are that day WILL come – so here's some advice about how to prepare for the joys of morning sickness. . .

- **Find out if you're immune to Rubella** (German measles). A simple blood test will tell you whether or not you're immune, and it's worth doing even if you think you've had it or you had the vaccination when you were at school. Rubella is usually a fairly mild disease, but it causes terrible damage to your baby if you get it in the early stages of pregnancy. If you aren't immune and get a rubella vaccination, you'll need to make sure you don't get pregnant for three months afterwards.

- **Start taking a vitamin called folic acid**. A dose of just 400 micrograms, available from the chemist, taken from before you conceive until you're 12 weeks pregnant, reduces your chance of having a baby with the spinal problem spina bifida by up to 75%.

- **Give up the fags**. You'll never have another incentive like it. It causes all sorts of problems to babies, starving them of oxygen and possibly making them addicted to nicotine.

- **Look at how much you're drinking**. There's lots of evidence that drinking more than 10 units a week can increase your chance of miscarriage and harm your baby's development. Most medics and scientists say that up to five units a week (one or two drinks once or twice a week) won't do your baby any harm – although it might reduce your chances of conceiving. The best idea is probably to do whatever stresses you out the least – if stopping completely is easy, it's the thing to do, but don't beat yourself up over the odd glass (as long as you stick to under five units a week).

- **Get in shape for pregnancy**. It's a really good idea to get your weight as close as possible to your ideal before you get pregnant. You're less likely to have complications like diabetes if you're not too overweight when you're pregnant. Just as importantly, it's impossible to know if you'll be forced to spend the entire first three months of pregnancy eating to ward off morning sickness and to stop you chucking up over your boss.

- **Get fit**. It's well worth getting fit before you get pregnant – not least because you're more likely to persevere with exercise when you resemble a beached whale if you're already in the habit. There's plenty of exercise you can do when you're pregnant, although it's worth getting advice from your gym or fitness instructor. Don't forget that labour is damned hard work, so the fitter you are, the better you'll cope. You're also likely to get back into shape quicker afterwards.

Index

Those page numbers which appear in **bold** represent the more major sections of text on any topic